McGraw-Hill's

Medical Translation Visual Phrasebook

Neil Bobenhouse, MHA, EMT-P

New York   Chicago   San Francisco   Lisbon   London   Madrid   Mexico City
Milan   New Delhi   San Juan   Seoul   Singapore   Sydney   Toronto

1 2 3 4 5 6 7 8 9 10 CTP/CTP 1 9 8 7 6 5 4 3 2

ISBN   978-0-07-180142-3
MHID   0-07-180142-1

e-ISBN   978-0-07-180143-0
e-MHID   0-07-180143-X

Library of Congress Control Number 2012943120

NOTICE

This book is not intended to provide medical advice or to substitute for the advice of a licensed medical professional, and readers should consult an appropriate medical practitioner for all matters relating to their health. Medicine is an ever-changing science. As new research and clinical experience broaden our knowledge, changes in treatment and drug therapy are required. The authors and the publisher of this work have checked with sources believed to be reliable in their efforts to provide information that is complete and generally in accord with the standards accepted at the time of publication. However, in view of the possibility of human error or changes in medical sciences, neither the authors nor the publisher nor any other party who has been involved in the preparation or publication of this work warrants that the information contained herein is in every respect accurate or complete, and they disclaim all responsibility for any errors or omissions or for the results obtained from use of the information contained in this work. Readers are encouraged to confirm the information contained herein with other sources. For example and in particular, readers are advised to check the product information sheet included in the package of each drug they plan to administer to be certain that any information contained in this work is accurate and that changes have not been made in the recommended dose or in the contraindications for administration.

Credits appear on page 121

McGraw-Hill products are available at special quantity discounts to use as premiums and sales promotions or for use in corporate training programs. To contact a representative, please e-mail us at bulksales@mcgraw-hill.com.

This book is printed on acid-free paper.

ABOUT THE PHRASEBOOK

McGraw-Hill's Medical Translation Visual Phrasebook is a communication aid specifically designed for EMTs, paramedics, nurses, physicians, and other healthcare providers who need to communicate with non-English-speaking patients. This book is a valuable bridge for healthcare providers to better understand their patients before proper translation services can be accessed. You do not need to know any language other than English to successfully use this book. All foreign language elements are presented with visual images or phrased as yes-no questions. Non-English speaking patients can point to the relevant images or respond to simple questions with a nod of the head or a simple "yes" or "no" in order to communicate essential information.

The twenty languages included in this book are the most commonly spoken foreign languages in the largest U.S. metropolitan areas according to U.S. Census data. Each language features five main sections: (acute) medical complaint, physical examination, previous medical history, obstetric, and procedural requests/statements to aid with examination. These assessments feature the most basic words and phrases that allow you to get essential information from patients.

As with any medical assessment, a subjective account must be considered with vital signs and other objective measures. THIS PHRASEBOOK IS NOT A DIAGNOSTIC DEVICE AND CANNOT DIAGNOSE MEDICAL CONDITIONS. THIS PHRASEBOOK IS STRICTLY A TRANSLATION AID. It must be understood that no translation is absolute and perfect. All translations were written with a general audience in mind.

HOW TO USE THIS PHRASEBOOK

There are many ways to use *McGraw-Hill's Medical Translation Visual Phrasebook*. To get started, follow these five steps:

1. Open up the table of contents and show the patient the list of languages featured in the book.

2. The patient should point to the relevant "I speak ..." statement that shows which language he or she speaks.

3. After determining the target language, turn to the section that has the assessment or content you need.

4. Point to each statement starting from the top and moving down. These statements instruct the patient to reply in yes or no answers (or otherwise). The translated statements appear next to the English translations.

5. Use the the phrasebook to assist with your patient assessment.

Table of Contents

TABLE OF CONTENTS

مرحباً، أنا موظفة مختصة بالصحة. وأنا لا أتكلم (العربية.)
Hello, I am a healthcare professional. I do not speak Arabic.

جاوبني بنعم أو لا فقط.
Respond to me only *yes* or *no*.

هل عندك؟
Do you have?

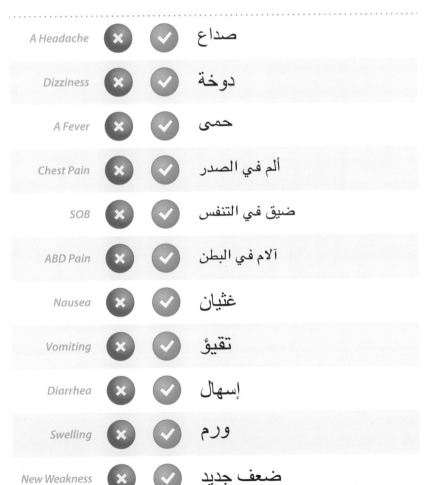

A Headache	✖	✔	صداع
Dizziness	✖	✔	دوخة
A Fever	✖	✔	حمى
Chest Pain	✖	✔	ألم في الصدر
SOB	✖	✔	ضيق في التنفس
ABD Pain	✖	✔	آلام في البطن
Nausea	✖	✔	غثيان
Vomiting	✖	✔	تقيؤ
Diarrhea	✖	✔	إسهال
Swelling	✖	✔	ورم
New Weakness	✖	✔	ضعف جديد

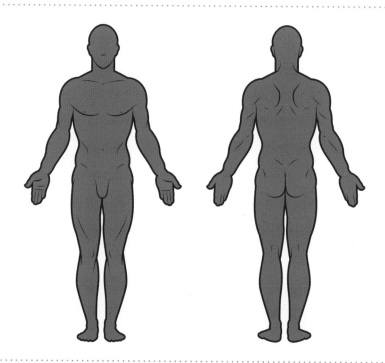
ARABIC / العربية

02

مرحباً، أنا موظفة مختصة بالصحة. وأنا لا أتكلم (العربية.)

Hello, I am a healthcare professional. I do not speak Arabic.

الرجاء أشر لي (على صورة هذا الشخص) أين الألم الذي عندك.

Please point (on this picture of a person) to where you have pain.

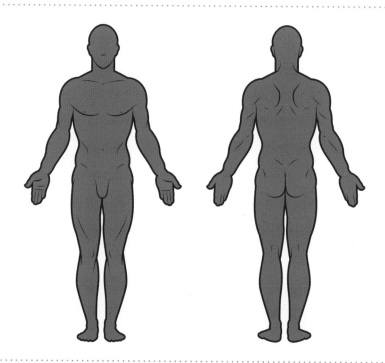

يرجى الإشارة على هذا المقياس إلى درجة الألم عندك.

Please point (on this scale) to rate your pain:

بدون ألم   ألم معتدل   ألم شديد

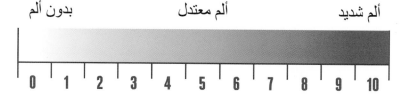

0   1   2   3   4   5   6   7   8   9   10

جاوبني بنعم أو لا فقط.

Do/Have you had: Respond to me only *yes* or *no*.

		Arabic
Rx Allergies?	✗ ✓	هل عندك حساسية من الأدوية؟
Asthma?	✗ ✓	هل عندك ربو؟
Hx of Ca?	✗ ✓	هل كان عندك سرطان بالماضي؟
CHF?	✗ ✓	هل عندك فشل القلب الإحتقاني؟
CRF?	✗ ✓	هل كان عندك فشل بالكلية في الماضي؟
CVA?	✗ ✓	هل أصابتك سكتة دماغية بأي وقت في الماضي؟
DM?	✗ ✓	هل عندك مرض السكري؟
Emphysema?	✗ ✓	هل عندك نفخة بالرئة؟
HIV/AIDS?	✗ ✓	هل عندك فيروس نقص المناعة أو مرض الإيدز؟
HTN?	✗ ✓	هل عندك إرتفاع بضغط الدم؟
An MI??	✗ ✓	هل أصابتك سكتة قلبية في الماضي؟
Psych Issues	✗ ✓	هل عندك أمراض نفسية؟
Recent Surgery?	✗ ✓	هل قمت بعملية جراحية حديثاً؟
Hx of Sz?	✗ ✓	هل أصابتك نوبات تشنجات في الماضي؟

ARABIC / العربية

04

مرحباً، أنا موظفة مختصة بالصحة. وأنا لا أتكلم (العربية.)

Hello, I am a healthcare professional. I do not speak Arabic.

جاوبني بنعم أو لا فقط.

Respond to me only *yes* or *no*.

Are you pregnant?	✗	✓	هل أنت حامل؟
Has your water broken?	✗	✓	هل تدفقت عليك مياه الولادة؟
Are you having contractions?	✗	✓	هل تشعرين بآلام تقلصات الولادة؟
Is the baby coming now?	✗	✓	هل سيخرج الطفل الآن؟
Do you have ABD pain?	✗	✓	هل تشعرين بآلام في البطن؟
Do you have vaginal pain?	✗	✓	هل تشعرين بآلام في المهبل؟
Do you have vaginal bleeding?	✗	✓	هل أنت تعاني من نزيف من المهبل؟
Do you have uncommon vaginal discharge?	✗	✓	هل عندك تدفق غير عادي من المهبل؟
Are you a high-risk pregnancy?	✗	✓	هل الحمل عندك مرتفع الخطورة؟
Have you had a recent physical injury?	✗	✓	هل كانت عندك إصابة جسدية حديثة؟
Have you had complications with a past pregnancy?	✗	✓	هل كانت عندك تعقيدات في الحمل السابق؟

الرجاء أعلمني عدد الأسابيع التي مرت منذ آخر دورة شهرية لديك.

Indicate how many weeks have passed since your last menstrual period.

<   1   2   3   4   5   6   7   8   9

كم شهرا مرت و أنت حامل.

Indicate how many months you have been pregnant.

<   1   2   3   4   5   6   7   8   9

أذكري الموعد المحدد لك للولادة؟

Indicate what date you are due to give birth.

1	2	3	4	5	6	7	سبتمبر/إيلول September	مايو/أيار May	يناير / كانون ثاني January
8	9	10	11	12	13	14	أكتوبر/تشرين أول October	يونيو/حزيران June	فبراير/شباط February
15	16	17	18	19	20	21	نوفمبر/تشرين ثاني November	يوليو/تموز July	مارس/آذار March
22	23	24	25	26	27	28	ديسمبر/كانون أول December	أغسطس/آب August	أبريل/نيسان April
29	30	31							

أشر لي كم مرة أصبحت حامل.

Indicate how many times you have been pregnant.

0   1   2   3   4   5   6   7   8   9

أشر لي كم عدد الأطفال الذي عندك.

Indicate how many children you have.

0   1   2   3   4   5   6   7   8   9

أشر لي كم مرة حدث عندك الإجهاض أو الإخفاق في الولادة.

Indicate how many abortions or miscarriages you have had.

0   1   2   3   4   5   6   7   8   9

ستحضر المترجمة قريبًا.
An interpreter will be here shortly.

يرجى التبول في الكوب. عند الإنتهاء ضعي الغطاء عليه وأعطه لي.
Please urinate in this cup. When you are finished, please attach the lid.

أحتاج لأن أضع لك إبرة في الوريد. يمكن أن تؤلمك قليلاً.
I need to start an IV. This may hurt a little.

أحتاج لأن أضع لك بعض اللصقات على صدرك لكي أفحص قلبك.
I need to put some stickers on your chest in order to examine your heart.

أحتاج لأن أضع لك أنبوبة قسطرة في المبولة. سيكون ذلك غير مريح.
I need to put a tube in your bladder. This will be uncomfortable.

أحتاج لأن أفحص رأسك ووجهك.
I need to examine your head and face.

إفتحي فمك من فضلك.
Please open your mouth.

أحتاج لأن أفحص صدرك، قلبك، ورئتيك.
I need to examine your chest, heart, and lungs.

أحتاج لأن أفحص بطنك. يمكن أن يكون ذلك غير مريح.
I need to examine your abdomen. Slight discomfort may occur.

أحتاج لأن أفحص الحوض والشرج. يمكن أن يكون ذلك غير مريح.
I need to examine your pelvis and rectum. Slight discomfort may occur.

سأعطيك دواء يمكن أن يجعلك تشعرين قليلاً بعدم الراحة.
I am going to give you a medication that may cause temporary discomfort.

سأعطيك دواء يمكن أن يجعلك تشعرين مؤقتًا بالنعاس أو بدوار في الرأس.
I am going to give you a medication that may make you feel sleepy or light-headed.

أنا سآخذك للحصول تصوير طبقي محوري. وهذا لن يؤلم.
I am going to take you to get a medical scan. This will not hurt.

Zdravo, ja sam zdravstveni radnik. Ja ne govorim Bosanski/Hrvatski/Srpski.
Hello, I am a healthcare professional. I do not speak Bosnian/Croatian/Serbian.

Molim vas da mi odgovorite sa da ili ne.
Respond to me only *yes* or *no*.

Da li imate?
Do you have?

Glavobolju	✓	✗	*A Headache*
Vrtoglavicu	✓	✗	*Dizziness*
Temperaturu	✓	✗	*A Fever*
Bol u grudima	✓	✗	*Chest Pain*
Problem sa disanjem	✓	✗	*SOB*
Bol u abdomenu	✓	✗	*ABD Pain*
Mučninu	✓	✗	*Nausea*
Povraćanje	✓	✗	*Vomiting*
Proljev	✓	✗	*Diarrhea*
Oticanje	✓	✗	*Swelling*
Dodatnu slabost	✓	✗	*New Weakness*

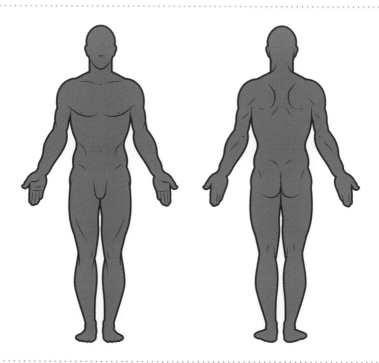
BOSNIAN/CROATIAN/SERBIAN /Bosanski/Hrvatski/Srpski

08

Zdravo, ja sam zdravstveni radnik. Ja ne govorim Bosanski/Hrvatski/Srpski.
Hello, I am a healthcare professional. I do not speak Bosnian/Croatian/Serbian.

Molim vas pokažite mi na ovoj slici gdje vas boli.
Please point (on this picture of a person) to where you have pain.

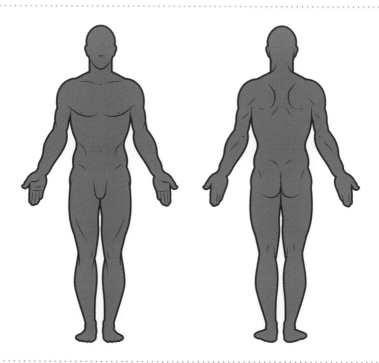

Molimo vas da nam pokažete (na ovoj skali) jačinu vašeg bola.
Please point (on this scale) to rate your pain.

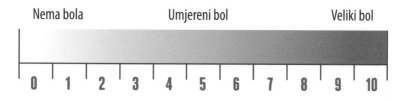

Nema bola	Umjereni bol	Veliki bol

0 1 2 3 4 5 6 7 8 9 10

Molim vas da mi odgovorite sa da ili ne.
Respond to me only *yes* or *no*.

Do/Have you had:

Da li imate alergije na lijekove?	✔ ✖	*Rx Allergies*
Da li imate astmu?	✔ ✖	*Asthma*
Da li imate istoriju raka?	✔ ✖	*Hx of Ca*
Da li imate kongenitalnu srčanu bolest?	✔ ✖	*CHF*
Da li imate istoriju poteškoća sa bubrezima?	✔ ✖	*CRF*
Da li ste ikada imali moždani udar?	✔ ✖	*CVA*
Da li imate šećernu bolest ili dijabetes?	✔ ✖	*DM*
Da li imate emfizem (Hronična opstrukcijska plućna bolest)	✔ ✖	*Emphysema*
Da li imate HIV ili Sidu?	✔ ✖	*HIV/AIDS*
Da li imate visok krvni pritisak?	✔ ✖	*HTN*
Da li ste imali srčani udar?	✔ ✖	*An MI*
Da li imate psiholoških problema?	✔ ✖	*Psych Issues*
Da li ste nedavno imali operaciju?	✔ ✖	*Recent Surgery*
Da li imate istoriju napada gubljenja svijesti?	✔ ✖	*Hx of Sz*

BOSNIAN/CROATIAN/SERBIAN /BOSANSKI/HRVATSKI/SRPSKI

10

Zdravo, ja sam zdravstveni radnik. Ja ne govorim Bosanski/Hrvatski/Srpski.
Hello, I am a healthcare professional. I do not speak Bosnian/Croatian/Serbian.

Molim vas da mi odgovorite sa da ili ne.
Respond to me only *yes* or *no*.

Da li ste trudni?	✔	✘	*Are you pregnant?*
Da li vam je pukla pukao vodenjak?	✔	✘	*Has your water broken?*
Da li imate trudove?	✔	✘	*Are you having contractions?*
Da li beba izlazi sada?	✔	✘	*Is the baby coming now?*
Da li imate bol u području abdomena?	✔	✘	*Do you have ABD pain?*
Da li imate vaginalni bol?	✔	✘	*Do you have vaginal pain?*
Da li imate vaginalno krvarenje?	✔	✘	*Do you have vaginal bleeding?*
Da li imate neoubičajeno vaginalno izlučivanje?	✔	✘	*Do you have uncommon vaginal discharge?*
Da li imate visokorizičnu trudnoću?	✔	✘	*Are you a high-risk pregnancy?*
Da li ste imali nedavnu fizičku povredu?	✔	✘	*Have you had a recent physical injury?*
Da li ste imali problema sa ranijim trudnoćama?	✔	✘	*Have you had complications with a past pregnancy?*

Koliko je prošlo sedmica od posljednje menstruacije?

Indicate how many weeks have passed since your last menstrual period.

< 1 2 3 4 5 6 7 8 9

Recite nam u kojem ste mjesecu trudnoce?

Indicate how many months you have been pregnant.

< 1 2 3 4 5 6 7 8 9

Navedite kada treba da se porodite.

Indicate the date you are due to give birth.

Januar	Maj	Septembar						
January	May	September	1	2	3	4	5	6	7
Februar	Juni	Oktobar	8	9	10	11	12	13	14
February	June	October	15	16	17	18	19	20	21
Mart	Juli	Novembar							
March	July	November	22	23	24	25	26	27	28
April	August	Decembar	29	30	31				
April	August	December							

Koliko puta ste bili trudni.

Indicate how many times you have been pregnant.

0 1 2 3 4 5 6 7 8 9

Koliko djece imate.

Indicate how many children you have.

0 1 2 3 4 5 6 7 8 9

Da li ste imali spontane pobačaje ili abortuse i koliko puta.

Indicate how many abortions or miscarriages you have had.

0 1 2 3 4 5 6 7 8 9

Prevodilac će uskoro doći.
An interpreter will be here shortly.

Molimo vas da nam date uzorak mokraće u ovoj šoljici. Kada završite, stavite poklopac i dajte nam šoljicu.
Please urinate in this cup. When you are finished, please attach the lid.

Moram početi da vam dajem infuziju. Ovo vas može malo zaboliti.
I need to start an IV. This may hurt a little.

Moram da stavim ove naljepnice na vaše grudi kako bi vam pregledali vaše srce.
I need to put some stickers on your chest in order to examine your heart.

Moram da stavim cijevčicu u vaš mokraćni mjehur. Ovo će biti neugodno.
I need to put a tube in your bladder. This will be uncomfortable.

Moram da vam pregledam glavu i lice.
I need to examine your head and face.

Molim vas da otvorite usta.
Please open your mouth.

Moram da pregledam vaš grudni koš, srce i pluća.
I need to examine your chest, heart, and lungs.

Moram da pregledam vaš abdomen. Pregled može biti neugodan.
I need to examine your abdomen. Slight discomfort may occur.

Moram pregledati pelvis i rektum. Pregled može biti neugodan.
I need to examine your pelvis and rectum. Slight discomfort may occur.

Dati ću vam lijekove koji vam privremeno mogu smetati.
I am going to give you a medication that may cause temporary discomfort.

Dati ću vam lijekove koji vas privremeno mogu učiniti pospanim ili izazvati da vam se vrti u glavi.
I am going to give you a medication that may make you feel sleepy or light-headed.

Odvesti ću vas da uraditi medicinski snimak. Ovo neće boljeti.
I am going to take you to get a medical scan. This will not hurt.

您好，我是一名健康护理专业人员。我不会说中文。
Hello, I am a healthcare professional. I do not speak Chinese.

您只需回答 是 或者 不是。
Respond to me only *yes* or *no*.

您有以下症状吗？
Do you have?

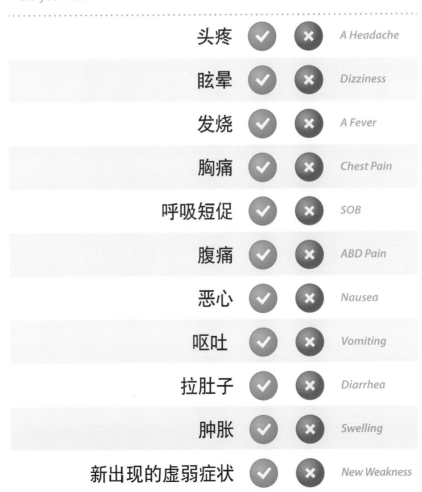

头疼	✓	✕	*A Headache*
眩晕	✓	✕	*Dizziness*
发烧	✓	✕	*A Fever*
胸痛	✓	✕	*Chest Pain*
呼吸短促	✓	✕	*SOB*
腹痛	✓	✕	*ABD Pain*
恶心	✓	✕	*Nausea*
呕吐	✓	✕	*Vomiting*
拉肚子	✓	✕	*Diarrhea*
肿胀	✓	✕	*Swelling*
新出现的虚弱症状	✓	✕	*New Weakness*

14

您好，我是一名健康护理专业人员。我不会说中文。
Hello, I am a healthcare professional. I do not speak Chinese.

请指出（用这张照片上的人）您什么地方疼。
Please point (on this picture of a person) to where you have pain.

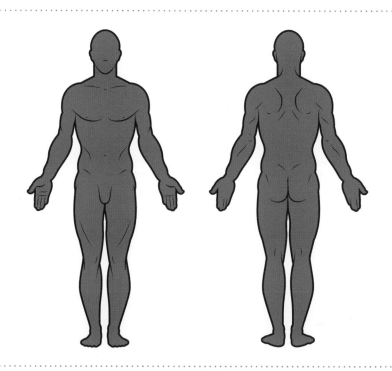

请（在下方标尺上）指出您的疼痛程度:
Please point (on this scale) to rate your pain:

无痛　　　　　　　中度疼痛　　　　　严重疼痛

0　1　2　3　4　5　6　7　8　9　10

您只需回答 是 或者 不是。
Respond to me only *yes* or *no*.

Do/Have you had:

您对某些药物过敏吗？   *Rx Allergies*

您有哮喘病吗？   *Asthma*

您有癌症病吗？   *Hx of Ca*

您有充血性心力衰吗？   *CHF*

您有肾衰竭病吗？   *CRF*

您患过中风吗？   *CVA*

您有糖尿病吗？   *DM*

您有肺气肿吗？   *Emphysema*

您有携带艾滋病病毒或患有艾滋病吗？   *HIV/AIDS*

您有高血压吗？   *HTN*

您有过心脏病发作吗？   *An MI*

您有心理问题吗？   *Psych Issues*

您最近动过手术吗？   *Recent Surgery*

您有癫痫病史吗？ *Hx of Sz*

CHINESE / 中文

16

您好，我是一名健康护理专业人员。我不会说中文。
Hello, I am a healthcare professional. I do not speak Chinese.

您只需回答 是 或者 不是。
Respond to me only *yes* or *no*.

您怀孕了吗？			*Are you pregnant?*
您的羊水破了吗？			*Has your water broken?*
您开始阵痛了吗？			*Are you having contractions?*
胎儿要出来了吗？			*Is the baby coming now?*
您的下腹痛吗？			*Do you have ABD pain?*
您的阴道痛吗？			*Do you have vaginal pain?*
您有阴道出血症状吗？			*Do you have vaginal bleeding?*
您的阴道排泄物不正常吗？			*Do you have uncommon vaginal discharge?*
您属于高危妊娠者吗？			*Are you a high-risk pregnancy?*
您最近身体受过伤吗？			*Have you had a recent physical injury?*
您过去怀孕期间有过任何并发症吗？			*Have you had complications with a past pregnancy?*

您好, 我是医务护理员。我不说中文。

Indicate how many weeks have passed since your last menstrual period.

<   1   2   3   4   5   6   7   8   9

请告诉我从您上次来月经到现在过了几个星期。

Indicate how many months you have been pregnant.

<   1   2   3   4   5   6   7   8   9

指出您的预产期:

Indicate what date you are due to give birth.

一月 January	五月 May	九月 September		1	2	3	4	5	6	7
二月 \February	六月 June	十月 October		8	9	10	11	12	13	14
三月 March	七月 July	十一月 November		15	16	17	18	19	20	21
四月 April	八月 August	十二月 December		22	23	24	25	26	27	28
				29	30	31				

请告诉我您怀过几次孕。

Indicate how many times you have been pregnant.

0   1   2   3   4   5   6   7   8   9

请告诉我您有几个孩子。

Indicate how many children you have.

0   1   2   3   4   5   6   7   8   9

请告诉我您有过几次人流或流产。

Indicate how many abortions or miscarriages you have had.

0   1   2   3   4   5   6   7   8   9

口译员很快就会过来。
An interpreter will be here shortly.

请在这个容器里小便。小便后请将容器盖子盖上，给我。
Please urinate in this cup. When you are finished, please attach the lid.

我需要给您做静脉注射，可能会有一点疼。
I need to start an IV. This may hurt a little.

为了检查您的心脏、我需要在您的胸上放些贴纸。
I need to put some stickers on your chest in order to examine your heart.

我需要在您的膀胱插一根试管，您会感到有些不舒服。
I need to put a tube in your bladder. This will be uncomfortable.

我需要检查您的头部和面部。
I need to examine your head and face.

请张开您的嘴。
Please open your mouth.

我需要检查您的胸腔、心脏和肺部。
I need to examine your chest, heart, and lungs.

我需要检查您的下腹，您可能会感到有些不舒服。
I need to examine your abdomen. Slight discomfort may occur.

我需要检查您的骨盆和直肠，您可能会感到有些不舒服。
I need to examine your pelvis and rectum. Slight discomfort may occur.

我会给您上药，您会感到短暂的不适。
I am going to give you a medication that may cause temporary discomfort.

我会给您上药，您会感到发困或头晕。
I am going to give you a medication that may make you feel sleepy or light-headed.

我会给您做一个无痛医疗扫描。
I am going to take you to get a medical scan. This will not hurt.

Bonjour, je suis un infirmier/infirmière/médecin. Je ne parle pas français.
Hello, I am a healthcare professional. I do not speak French.

Répondez-moi uniquement par oui ou par non.
Respond to me only *yes* or *no*.

Souffrez-vous de?
Do you have?

Maux de tête	✓	✗	*A Headache*
Vertiges	✓	✗	*Dizziness*
Fièvre	✓	✗	*A Fever*
Douleurs thoraciques	✓	✗	*Chest Pain*
Essoufflements	✓	✗	*SOB*
Maux de ventre	✓	✗	*ABD Pain*
Nausées	✓	✗	*Nausea*
Vomissements	✓	✗	*Vomiting*
Diarrhée	✓	✗	*Diarrhea*
Gonflements	✓	✗	*Swelling*
Faiblesse	✓	✗	*New Weakness*

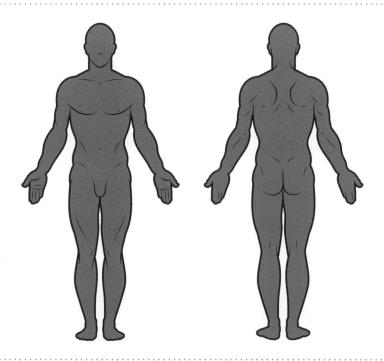

FRENCH / Français

20

Bonjour, je suis un infirmier/infirmière/médecin. Je ne parle pas français.

Hello, I am a healthcare professional. I do not speak French.

Pouvez-vous indiquer (sur cette photo) où vous avez mal?

Please point (on this picture of a person) to where you have pain.

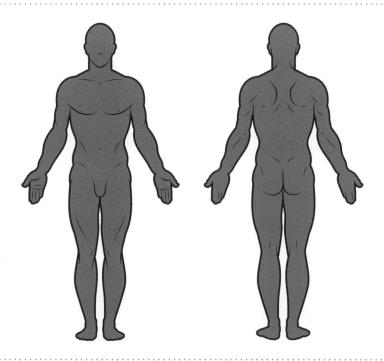

Indiquez l'intensité de la douleur que vous ressentez sur l'échelle suivante :

Please point (on this scale) to rate your pain:

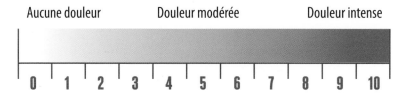

Répondez-moi uniquement par oui ou par non.
Respond to me only *yes* or *no*.

Do/Have you had:

Etes-vous allergique à des médicaments?	✓	✗	*Rx Allergies*
Souffrez-vous d'asthme?	✓	✗	*Asthma*
Avez-vous des antécédents de cancer dans votre famille?	✓	✗	*Hx of Ca*
Souffrez-vous d'insuffisance cardiaque congestive?	✓	✗	*CHF*
Avez-vous des antécédents d'insuffisance rénale dans votre famille?	✓	✗	*CRF*
Avez-vous déjà eu un accident vasculaire cérébral?	✓	✗	*CVA*
Souffrez-vous de diabète?	✓	✗	*DM*
Souffrez-vous d'emphysème?	✓	✗	*Emphysema*
Etes-vous porteur du VIH ou souffrez-vous du SIDA?	✓	✗	*HIV/AIDS*
Faites-vous de l'hypertension?	✓	✗	*HTN*
Avez-vous déjà fait une crise cardiaque?	✓	✗	*An MI*
Souffrez-vous de problèmes psychologiques?	✓	✗	*Psych Issues*
Avez-vous récemment été opéré(e)?	✓	✗	*Recent Surgery*
Avez-vous des antécédents épileptiques dans votre famille?	✓	✗	*Hx of Sz*

FRENCH / Français

22

Bonjour, je suis un infirmier/infirmière/médecin. Je ne parle pas français.
Hello, I am a healthcare professional. I do not speak French.

Répondez-moi uniquement par oui ou par non.
Respond to me only *yes* or *no*.

Etes-vous enceinte?	✓	✗	Are you pregnant?
Avez-vous perdu les eaux?	✓	✗	Has your water broken?
Avez-vous des contractions?	✓	✗	Are you having contractions?
Sentez-vous venir le bébé?	✓	✗	Is the baby coming now?
Souffrez-vous de douleurs abdominales?	✓	✗	Do you have ABD pain?
Souffrez-vous de douleurs vaginales?	✓	✗	Do you have vaginal pain?
Avez-vous des saignements vaginaux?	✓	✗	Do you have vaginal bleeding?
Avez-vous des pertes vaginales inhabituelles?	✓	✗	Do you have uncommon vaginal discharge?
Votre grossesse est-elle à haut risque?	✓	✗	Are you a high-risk pregnancy?
Avez-vous récemment été blessée?	✓	✗	Have you had a recent physical injury?
Avez-vous souffert de complications lors de votre grossesse précédente?	✓	✗	Have you had complications with a past pregnancy?

Indiquez à combien de semaines remontent vos dernières règles.
Indicate how many weeks have passed since your last menstrual period.

<   1   2   3   4   5   6   7   8   9

Indiquez de combien de mois vous êtes enceinte.
Indicate how many months you have been pregnant.

<   1   2   3   4   5   6   7   8   9

Veuillez indiquer la date prévue de votre accouchement.
Indicate what date you are due to give birth.

Janvier	Mai	Septembre	1	2	3	4	5	6	7
January	May	September							
Février	Juin	Octobre	8	9	10	11	12	13	14
February	June	October							
			15	16	17	18	19	20	21
Mars	Juillet	Novembre							
March	July	November	22	23	24	25	26	27	28
Avril	Août	Décembre	29	30	31				
April	August	December							

Combien de fois avez-vous été enceinte?
Indicate how many times you have been pregnant.

0   1   2   3   4   5   6   7   8   9

Combien d'enfants avez-vous?
Indicate how many children you have.

0   1   2   3   4   5   6   7   8   9

Combien d'avortements avez-vous eus, ou combien de fausses couches avez-vous faites ?
Indicate how many abortions or miscarriages you have had.

0   1   2   3   4   5   6   7   8   9

24

Un traducteur nous rejoindra bientôt.
An interpreter will be here shortly.

Veuillez uriner dans ce gobelet.
Lorsque vous aurez terminé, mettez le couvercle en place.
Please urinate in this cup. When you are finished, please attach the lid.

Je dois commencer une IV. Ce sera peut-être un peu douloureux.
I need to start an IV. This may hurt a little.

Je dois mettre des autocollants sur votre poitrine pour examiner votre cœur.
I need to put some stickers on your chest in order to examine your heart.

Je dois mettre un tube dans votre vessie. Cela pourra être désagréable.
I need to put a tube in your bladder. This will be uncomfortable.

Je dois examiner votre tête et votre visage.
I need to examine your head and face.

Veillez ouvrir la bouche.
Please open your mouth.

Je dois examiner votre gorge, votre cœur et vos poumons.
I need to examine your chest, heart, and lungs.

Je dois examiner votre abdomen. Cela peut être désagréable.
I need to examine your abdomen. Slight discomfort may occur.

Je dois examiner votre bassin et votre rectum. Cela peut être désagréable.
I need to examine your pelvis and rectum. Slight discomfort may occur.

Je vais vous donner un médicament qui pourra vous être désagréable pendant quelques temps.
I am going to give you a medication that may cause temporary discomfort.

Je vais vous donner un médicament qui pourra vous rendre somnolent ou vous donner des vertiges.
I am going to give you a medication that may make you feel sleepy or light-headed.

Je vais vous emmener passer un scanner. Cela n'est pas douloureux.
I am going to take you to get a medical scan. This will not hurt.

Guten Tag, ich bin Krankenschwester / Krankenpfleger / Arzt / Ärztin.
Ich spreche kein Deutsch.
Hello, I am a healthcare professional. I do not speak German.

Antworten Sie mir bitte nur mit ja oder nein.
Respond to me only *yes* or *no*.

Haben Sie einen der folgenden Zustände?
Do you have?

Kopfschmerzen	✓	✗	*A Headache*
Schwindel	✓	✗	*Dizziness*
Fieber	✓	✗	*A Fever*
Brustschmerzen	✓	✗	*Chest Pain*
Atemnot	✓	✗	*SOB*
Magenschmerzen	✓	✗	*ABD Pain*
Übelkeit	✓	✗	*Nausea*
Erbrechen	✓	✗	*Vomiting*
Diarrhöe / dünnflüssigen Stuhl	✓	✗	*Diarrhea*
Schwellungen	✓	✗	*Swelling*
Neu eingetretenes Schwächegefühl	✓	✗	*New Weakness*

GERMAN / DEUTSCH

Guten Tag, ich bin Krankenschwester / Krankenpfleger / Arzt / Ärztin.
Ich spreche kein Deutsch.

Hello, I am a healthcare professional. I do not speak German.

Bitte zeigen Sie mir (auf diesem Bild mit einem Menschen), wo es Ihnen wehtut.

Please point (on this picture of a person) to where you have pain.

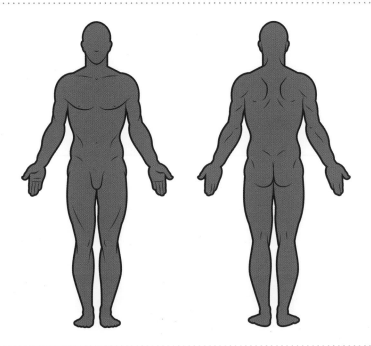

Bitte zeigen Sie auf diese Tafel, um Ihren Grad an Schmerzen anzuzeigen.

Please point (on this scale) to rate your pain:

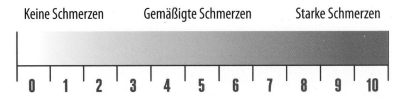

Keine Schmerzen   Gemäßigte Schmerzen   Starke Schmerzen

0   1   2   3   4   5   6   7   8   9   10

Antworten Sie mir bitte nur mit ja oder nein.
Respond to me only *yes* or *no*. Do/Have you had:

Sind Sie gegen bestimmte Arzneimittel allergisch?	✔	✖	*Rx Allergies*
Haben Sie Asthma?	✔	✖	*Asthma*
Haben oder hatten Sie oder ein Familienmitgleid Krebs?	✔	✖	*Hx of Ca*
Leiden Sie unter Herzinsuffizienz?	✔	✖	*CHF*
Litten Sie schon einmal unter Nierenversagen?	✔	✖	*CRF*
Hatten Sie schon einmal einen Schlaganfall?	✔	✖	*CVA*
Haben Sie Diabetes?	✔	✖	*DM*
Leiden Sie unter Lungenemphysem?	✔	✖	*Emphysema*
Sind Sie Träger des HI-Virus oder haben Sie AIDS?	✔	✖	*HIV/AIDS*
Leiden Sie unter Bluthochdruck?	✔	✖	*HTN*
Hatten Sie schon einmal einen Herzinfarkt?	✔	✖	*An MI*
Leiden Sie unter psychischen Problemen?	✔	✖	*Psych Issues*
Wurden Sie in letzter Zeit operiert?	✔	✖	*Recent Surgery*
Hatten Sie schon einmal Krampfanfälle?	✔	✖	*Hx of Sz*

Guten Tag, ich bin Krankenschwester / Krankenpfleger / Arzt / Ärztin.
Ich spreche kein Deutsch.
Hello, I am a healthcare professional. I do not speak German.

Antworten Sie mir bitte nur mit ja oder nein.
Respond to me only *yes* or *no*.

Sind Sie schwanger?	✓	✗	Are you pregnant?
Ist die Fruchtblase geplatzt?	✓	✗	Has your water broken?
Haben die Wehen eingesetzt?	✓	✗	Are you having contractions?
Kommt das Baby jetzt?	✓	✗	Is the baby coming now?
Haben Sie Schmerzen im Unterleib?	✓	✗	Do you have ABD pain?
Haben Sie Schmerzen in der Scheide?	✓	✗	Do you have vaginal pain?
Blutet es bei Ihnen aus der Scheide?	✓	✗	Do you have vaginal bleeding?
Tritt bei Ihnen ein ungewöhnlicher Ausfluss aus der Scheide auf?	✓	✗	Do you have uncommon vaginal discharge?
Ist Ihre Schwangerschaft sehr riskant?	✓	✗	Are you a high-risk pregnancy?
Haben Sie sich kürzlich verletzt?	✓	✗	Have you had a recent physical injury?
Traten bei einer früheren Schwangerschaft Komplikationen auf?	✓	✗	Have you had complications with a past pregnancy?

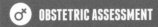
Wie viele Wochen ist es her, seitdem Sie Ihre letzte Regel gehabt haben?

Indicate how many weeks have passed since your last menstrual period.

< 1 2 3 4 5 6 7 8 9

Wie viele Monate sind Sie schwanger?

Indicate how many months you have been pregnant.

< 1 2 3 4 5 6 7 8 9

Nennen Sie uns bitte den Monat, in dem Sie gebären werden.

Indicate what date you are due to give birth.

Januar January	Mai May	September September	1	2	3	4	5	6	7
Februar February	Juni June	Oktober October	8	9	10	11	12	13	14
			15	16	17	18	19	20	21
März March	Juli July	November November	22	23	24	25	26	27	28
April April	August August	Dezember December	29	30	31				

Wie oft sind Sie schon schwanger gewesen?

Indicate how many times you have been pregnant.

0 1 2 3 4 5 6 7 8 9

Wie viele Kinder haben Sie?

Indicate how many children you have.

0 1 2 3 4 5 6 7 8 9

Wie viele Abtreibungen oder Fehlgeburten haben Sie gehabt?

Indicate how many abortions or miscarriages you have had.

0 1 2 3 4 5 6 7 8 9

Gleich kommt ein(e) Dolmetscher(in).
An interpreter will be here shortly.

Bitte urinieren Sie in diesen Becher. Danach verschließen Sie ihn bitte und geben Sie ihn mir.
Please urinate in this cup. When you are finished, please attach the lid.

Ich muss Ihnen eine intravenöse Kanüle legen. Möglicherweise tut es ein bisschen weh.
I need to start an IV. This may hurt a little.

Ich muss einige Applikatoren auf Ihrem Brustkorb aufbringen, um Ihr Herz abzuhören.
I need to put some stickers on your chest in order to examine your heart.

Ich muss einen Schlauch in Ihre Blase schieben. Das wird unangenehm sein.
I need to put a tube in your bladder. This will be uncomfortable.

Ich muss Ihren Kopf und Ihr Gesicht untersuchen.
I need to examine your head and face.

Bitte öffnen Sie Ihren Mund.
Please open your mouth.

Ich muss Ihre Brust, Ihr Herz und Ihre Lunge untersuchen.
I need to examine your chest, heart, and lungs.

Ich muss Ihren Unterleib untersuchen. Das kann unangenehm sein.
I need to examine your abdomen. Slight discomfort may occur.

Ich muss Ihr Becken und Ihr Rektum untersuchen. Das kann unangenehm sein.
I need to examine your pelvis and rectum. Slight discomfort may occur.

Ich gebe Ihnen jetzt ein Medikament, das zu kurzem Unbehagen führen kann.
I am going to give you a medication that may cause temporary discomfort.

Ich gebe Ihnen jetzt ein Medikament, das Sie schläfrig oder benommen machen kann.
I am going to give you a medication that may make you feel sleepy or light-headed.

Ich nehme Sie mit, um eine medizinische Aufnahme zu machen. Es wird nicht wehtun.
I am going to take you to get a medical scan. This will not hurt.

Γεια σας. Εργάζομαι στο χώρο της υγείας. Δεν μιλώ ελληνικά.
Hello, I am a healthcare professional. I do not speak Greek.

Απαντήστε μου μόνο με ναι ή όχι.
Respond to me only *yes* or *no*.

Εμφανίζετε;
Do you have?

Πονοκέφαλο	✓	✗	A Headache
Ζαλάδα	✓	✗	Dizziness
Πυρετό	✓	✗	A Fever
Πόνο στο στήθος	✓	✗	Chest Pain
Δυσκολία στην αναπνοή	✓	✗	SOB
Πόνο στην κοιλιά	✓	✗	ABD Pain
Ναυτία	✓	✗	Nausea
Τάση για έμετο	✓	✗	Vomiting
Διάρροια	✓	✗	Diarrhea
Πρήξιμο	✓	✗	Swelling
Κάποια αδυναμία που αισθάνεστε για πρώτη φορά	✓	✗	New Weakness

Γεια σας. Εργάζομαι στο χώρο της υγείας. Δεν μιλώ ελληνικά.
Hello, I am a healthcare professional. I do not speak Greek.

Παρακαλώ δείξτε (στην εικόνα με το ανθρώπινο σώμα) το σημείο όπου πονάτε.
Please point (on this picture of a person) to where you have pain.

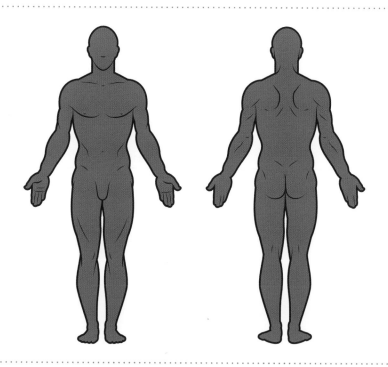

Παρακαλώ δείξτε (σ' αυτή την κλίμακα) πώς αξιολογείτε τον πόνο σας.
Please point (on this scale) to rate your pain:

Καθόλου πόνος   Μέτριος πόνος   Ισχυρός πόνος

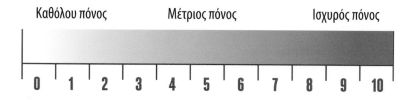

0 1 2 3 4 5 6 7 8 9 10

Απαντήστε μου μόνο με ναι ή όχι.
Respond to me only *yes* or *no*.   *Do/Have you had:*

Έχετε αλλεργίες σε φάρμακα;   *Rx Allergies*

Έχετε άσθμα;   *Asthma*

Είχατε ποτέ καρκίνο;   *Hx of Ca*

Έχετε συμφορητική καρδιακή ανεπάρκεια;   *CHF*

Είχατε ποτέ νεφρική ανεπάρκεια; *CRF*

Είχατε ποτέ εγκεφαλικό επεισόδιο;   *CVA*

Έχετε διαβήτη;   *DM*

Έχετε εμφύσημα; *Emphysema*

Είστε φορέας HIV ή έχετε τον ιό του AIDS;   *HIV/AIDS*

Έχετε υψηλή πίεση;   *HTN*

Είχατε ποτέ καρδιακή προσβολή;   *An MI*

Έχετε ψυχολογικά προβλήματα; *Psych Issues*

Εγχειριστήκατε πρόσφατα;   *Recent Surgery*

Είχατε ποτέ επιληπτικές κρίσεις;   *Hx of Sz*

Γεια σας. Εργάζομαι στο χώρο της υγείας. Δεν μιλώ ελληνικά.
Hello, I am a healthcare professional. I do not speak Greek.

Απαντήστε μου μόνο με ναι ή όχι.
Respond to me only *yes* or *no*.

Είστε έγκυος;			*Are you pregnant?*
Έχουν σπάσει τα νερά σας;			*Has your water broken?*
Έχετε συσπάσεις της μήτρας;			*Are you having contractions?*
Το μωρό έρχεται τώρα;			*Is the baby coming now?*
Έχετε πόνο στην κοιλιά;			*Do you have ABD pain?*
Έχετε κολπικό πόνο;			*Do you have vaginal pain?*
Έχετε κολπική αιμορραγία;			*Do you have vaginal bleeding?*
Έχετε ασυνήθιστες κολπικές εκκρίσεις;			*Do you have uncommon vaginal discharge?*
Έχετε εγκυμοσύνη υψηλού κινδύνου;			*Are you a high-risk pregnancy?*
Έχετε υποστεί πρόσφατα κάποιο τραυματισμό;			*Have you had a recent physical injury?*
Είχατε επιπλοκές σε προηγούμενη εγκυμοσύνη;			*Have you had complications with a past pregnancy?*

Αναφέρετε πόσες εβδομάδες έχουν περάσει από την τελευταία σας περίοδο.

Indicate how many weeks have passed since your last menstrual period.

< 1 2 3 4 5 6 7 8 9

Αναφέρετε σε ποιον μήνα της εγκυμοσύνης βρίσκεστε.

Indicate how many months you have been pregnant.

< 1 2 3 4 5 6 7 8 9

Αναφέρετε την ημερομηνία που περιμένετε να γεννήσετε.

Indicate what date you are due to give birth.

Ιανουάριος January	Μάιος May	Σεπτέμβριος September	1 2 3 4 5 6 7
Φεβρουάριος February	Ιούνιος June	Οκτώβριος October	8 9 10 11 12 13 14
Μάρτιος March	Ιούλιος July	Νοέμβριος November	15 16 17 18 19 20 21
			22 23 24 25 26 27 28
Απρίλιος April	Αύγουστος August	Δεκέμβριος December	29 30 31

Αναφέρετε πόσες φορές έχετε μείνει έγκυος.

Indicate how many times you have been pregnant.

0 1 2 3 4 5 6 7 8 9

Αναφέρετε πόσα παιδιά έχετε γεννήσει.

Indicate how many children you have delivered.

0 1 2 3 4 5 6 7 8 9

Αναφέρετε πόσες φορές έχετε κάνει έκτρωση ή έχετε αποβάλει.

Indicate how many abortions or miscarriages you have had.

0 1 2 3 4 5 6 7 8 9

Ένας διερμηνέας θα έρθει εδώ σύντομα.
An interpreter will be here shortly.

Παρακαλώ ουρήστε μέσα σ'αυτό το κύπελο. Όταν τελειώσετε, παρακαλώ τοποθετήστε το καπάκι και δώστε μου το κύπελο.
Please urinate in this cup. When you are finished, please attach the lid.

Χρειάζεται να ξεκινήσουμε ορό. Μπορεί να πονέσετε λίγο.
I need to start an IV. This may hurt a little.

Χρειάζεται να τοποθετήσω μερικά αυτοκόλλητα στο στήθος σας για να εξετάσω την καρδιά σας.
I need to put some stickers on your chest in order to examine your heart.

Χρειάζεται να τοποθετήσω ένα σωληνάκι στην ουροδόχο κύστη σας. Θα νιώσετε μια ενόχληση.
I need to put a tube in your bladder. This will be uncomfortable.

Χρειάζεται να εξετάσω το κεφάλι και το πρόσωπό σας.
I need to examine your head and face.

Παρακαλώ ανοίξτε το στόμα σας.
Please open your mouth.

Χρειάζεται να εξετάσω το στήθος, την καρδιά και τους πνεύμονές σας.
I need to examine your chest, heart, and lungs.

Χρειάζεται να εξετάσω την κοιλιά σας. Μπορεί να νιώσετε μια ενόχληση.
I need to examine your abdomen. Slight discomfort may occur.

Χρειάζεται να εξετάσω τη λεκάνη σας και τον πρωκτό σας. Μπορεί να νιώσετε μια ενόχληση.
I need to examine your pelvis and rectum. Slight discomfort may occur.

Θα σας δώσω ένα φάρμακο που είναι πιθανό να σας προκαλέσει προσωρινή ενόχληση.
I am going to give you a medication that may cause temporary discomfort.

Θα σας δώσω ένα φάρμακο που είναι πιθανό να σας φέρει προσωρινή υπηλία ή ελαφριά ζαλάδα.
I am going to give you a medication that may make you feel sleepy or light-headed.

Θα σας υποβάλω σε τομογραφία. Δεν θα πονέσετε.
I am going to take you to get a medical scan. This will not hurt.

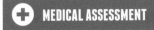
Bonjou, mwen se yon pwofesyonèl swen sante. Mwen pa pale Kreyòl Ayisyen.
Hello, I am a healthcare professional. I do not speak Haitian Creole.

Reponn mwen sèlman wi oswa non.
Respond to me only *yes* or *no*.

Èske ou gen?
Do you have?

Maltèt	✓	✗	*A Headache*
Tèt Vire	✓	✗	*Dizziness*
Lafyèv	✓	✗	*A Fever*
Doulè nan pwatrin	✓	✗	*Chest Pain*
Souf kout	✓	✗	*SOB*
Doulè nan vant	✓	✗	*ABD Pain*
Kèplen	✓	✗	*Nausea*
Vomisman	✓	✗	*Vomiting*
Dyare	✓	✗	*Diarrhea*
Anflamasyon	✓	✗	*Swelling*
Nouvo feblès	✓	✗	*New Weakness*

Bonjou, mwen se yon pwofesyonèl swen sante. Mwen pa pale Kreyòl Ayisyen.
Hello, I am a healthcare professional. I do not speak Haitian Creole.

Tanpri pwente ak dwèt ou (sou foto moun sa a) pou montre ki kote ou gen doulè.
Please point (on this picture of a person) to where you have pain.

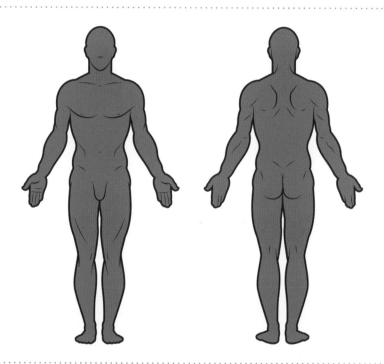

Tanpri pwente ak dwèt ou (sou echèl/imaj sa a) pou evalye doulè w.
Please point (on this scale) to rate your pain:

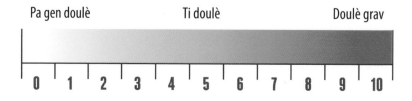

Pa gen doulè	Ti doulè	Doulè grav

0 1 2 3 4 5 6 7 8 9 10

Reponn mwen sèlman wi oswa non.
Respond to me only yes or no.   *Do/Have you had:*

Èske ou fè alèji ak medikaman?	✓ ✕	*Rx Allergies*
Èske ou soufri opresyon (las)?	✓ ✕	*Asthma*
Èske ou te gen antesedan kansè?	✓ ✕	*Hx of Ca*
Èske ou gen ensifizans kadyak konjestif?	✓ ✕	*CHF*
Èske ou gen antesedan ensifizans renal (nan ren)?	✓ ✕	*CRF*
Èske ou janm fè yon estwòk?	✓ ✕	*CVA*
Èske ou soufri dyabèt (ou fè sik)?	✓ ✕	*DM*
Èske ou gen anfizèm?	✓ ✕	*Emphysema*
Èske ou gen VIH oswa SIDA?	✓ ✕	*HIV/AIDS*
Èske ou soufri ipètansyon (tansyon ki wo)?	✓ ✕	*HTN*
Èske ou janm fè yon kriz kadyak?	✓ ✕	*An MI*
Èske ou gen pwoblèm sikolojik?	✓ ✕	*Psych Issues*
Èske ou fè yon operasyon pa gen lontan?	✓ ✕	*Recent Surgery*
Èske ou gen antesedan kriz malkadi?	✓ ✕	*Hx of Sz*

Bonjou, mwen se yon pwofesyonèl swen sante. Mwen pa pale Kreyòl Ayisyen.
Hello, I am a healthcare professional. I do not speak Haitian Creole.

Reponn mwen sèlman wi oswa non.
Respond to me only *yes* or *no*.

Èske ou ansent?	✓ ✗	Are you pregnant?
Èske ou kase lèzo?	✓ ✗	Has your water broken?
Èske ou gen kontraksyon?	✓ ✗	Are you having contractions?
Èske tibebe a ap sòti kounye a?	✓ ✗	Is the baby coming now?
Èske ou gen doulè nan abdomèn (nan vant)?	✓ ✗	Do you have ABD pain?
Èske ou gen doulè nan vajen?	✓ ✗	Do you have vaginal pain?
Èske ou gen senyman nan vajen?	✓ ✗	Do you have vaginal bleeding?
Èske ou gen sekresyon nan vajen ki pa nòmal?	✓ ✗	Do you have uncommon vaginal discharge?
Èske ou gen yon gwosès ki gen risk elve?	✓ ✗	Are you a high-risk pregnancy?
Èske ou te gen yon domaj fizik (nan kò w) sa pa fè lontan?	✓ ✗	Have you had a recent physical injury?
Èske ou te gen konplikasyon avèk yon gwosès anvan sa?	✓ ✗	Have you had complications with a past pregnancy?

Konbyen semenn ki deja pase depi dènye fwa ou te gen règ ou.

Indicate how many weeks have passed since your last menstrual period.

<   1   2   3   4   5   6   7   8   9

Konbyen mwa gwosès ou genyen.

Indicate how many months you have been pregnant.

<   1   2   3   4   5   6   7   8   9

- -

Bay dat ou sipoze akouche a.

Indicate what date you are due to give birth.

Janvye	Me	Septanm							
January	May	September	1	2	3	4	5	6	7
Fevriye	Jen	Oktòb	8	9	10	11	12	13	14
February	June	October	15	16	17	18	19	20	21
Mas	Jiyè	Novanm							
March	July	November	22	23	24	25	26	27	28
Avril	Out	Desanm	29	30	31				
April	August	December							

- -

Konbyen fwa ou te ansent deja.

Indicate how many times you have been pregnant.

0   1   2   3   4   5   6   7   8   9

Konbyen timoun ou akouche deja.

Indicate how many children you have delivered.

0   1   2   3   4   5   6   7   8   9

Konbyen avòtman oswa foskouch ou fè deja.

Indicate how many abortions or miscarriages you have had.

0   1   2   3   4   5   6   7   8   9

- -

Ap gen yon tradiktè kap vini talè
An interpreter will be here shortly.

Tanpri, pipi nan gode sa a. Lè w fini tanpri bouche l ak bouchon an epi remèt mwen gode a.
Please urinate in this cup. When you are finished, please attach the lid.

Mwen bezwen mete sewòm nan. Ou ka santi yon ti doulè.
I need to start an IV. This may hurt a little.

Mwen bezwen mete kèk otokolan sou pwatrin ou pou nou sa egzamine kè w.
I need to put some stickers on your chest in order to examine your heart.

Mwen bezwen mete yon tib nan blad pipi w. Sa pral fè w santi w malalèz.
I need to put a tube in your bladder. This will be uncomfortable.

Mwen bezwen egzamine tèt ou ak figi w.
I need to examine your head and face.

Tanpri ouvri bouch ou.
Please open your mouth.

Mwen bezwen egzamine pwatrin ou, kè w ak poumon w yo.
I need to examine your chest, heart, and lungs.

Mwen bezwen egzamine abdomèn (vant) ou. Sa ka fè w santi w malalèz.
I need to examine your abdomen. Slight discomfort may occur.

Mwen bezwen egzamine basen w ak twou dèyè w. Sa ka fè w santi w malalèz.
I need to examine your pelvis and rectum. Slight discomfort may occur.

Mwen pral ba w yon medikaman ki pral fè w santi w malalèz pandan yon timoman.
I am going to give you a medication that may cause temporary discomfort.

Mwen pral ba w yon medikaman ki ka fè w anvi dòmi oswa gen tèt vire pandan yon timoman.
I am going to give you a medication that may make you feel sleepy or light-headed.

Map mennen w pou w al fè yon eskanografi medikal. Li pap fè w mal ditou.
I am going to take you to get a medical scan. This will not hurt.

שלום, אני מטפל/ת מקצועי/ת. איני דובר/ת שפה.
Hello, I am a healthcare professional. I do not speak Hebrew.

ענה/י לי רק בכן או לא.
Respond to me only *yes* or *no*.

האם יש לך?
Do you have?

A Headache	✖	✔	כאב ראש
Dizziness	✖	✔	סחרחורת
A Fever	✖	✔	חום
Chest Pain	✖	✔	כאבים בחזה
SOB	✖	✔	קוצר נשימה
ABD Pain	✖	✔	כאב בטן
Nausea	✖	✔	בחילה
Vomiting	✖	✔	הקאות
Diarrhea	✖	✔	שלשול
Swelling	✖	✔	נפיחות
New Weakness	✖	✔	חולשה חדשה

שלום, אני מטפל/ת מקצועי/ת. איני דובר/ת שפה.

Hello, I am a healthcare professional. I do not speak Hebrew.

נא להצביע (בתמונה הזו של בן אדם) על המקום שכואב לך.

Please point (on this picture of a person) to where you have pain.

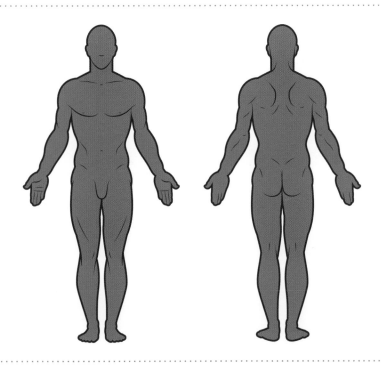

נא לסמן (בסרגל זה) את דירוג את הכאב שלך.

Please point (on this scale) to rate your pain:

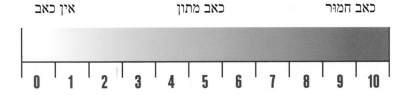

אין כאב	כאב מתון	כאב חמור

0 1 2 3 4 5 6 7 8 9 10

ענה/י לי רק בכן או לא.

Do/Have you had: Respond to me only *yes* or *no*.

Rx Allergies	✖ ✔	?האם יש לך רגישויות לתרופות
Asthma	✖ ✔	?האם יש לך אסתמה
Hx of Ca	✖ ✔	?האם יש לך היסטוריה של סרטן
CHF	✖ ✔	?האם יש לך אי-ספיקת לב מוגדש
CRF	✖ ✔	?האם יש לך היסטוריה של אי-ספיקת כליות
CVA	✖ ✔	?האם היה לך אי-פעם שבץ
DM	✖ ✔	?האם יש לך סוכרת
Emphysema	✖ ✔	?(האם יש לך נפחת (אמפיזמה
HIV/AIDS	✖ ✔	האם אתה נושא את נגיף הכשל החיסוני האנושי או חולה באיידס?
HTN	✖ ✔	?האם יש לך יתר לחץ דם
An MI	✖ ✔	?האם היה לך התקף לב
Psych Issues	✖ ✔	?האם יש לך בעיות פסיכולוגיות
Recent Surgery	✖ ✔	?האם עברת ניתוח לאחרונה
Hx of Sz	✖ ✔	?האם יש לך היסטוריה של התקפים אפילפטיים

שלום, אני מטפל/ת מקצועי/ת. איני דובר/ת שפה.
Hello, I am a healthcare professional. I do not speak Hebrew.

ענה/י לי רק בכן או לא.
Respond to me only *yes* or *no*.

Are you pregnant?	✖	✔	האם את בהריון?
Has your water broken?	✖	✔	האם הייתה לך ירידת מים?
Are you having contractions?	✖	✔	האם יש לך צירים?
Is the baby coming now?	✖	✔	האם התינוק עומד להיוולד עכשיו?
Do you have ABD pain?	✖	✔	האם יש לך כאב בטן?
Do you have vaginal pain?	✖	✔	האם יש לך כאבים בנרתיק?
Do you have vaginal bleeding?	✖	✔	האם יש לך דימום מהנרתיק?
Do you have uncommon vaginal discharge?	✖	✔	האם יש לך הפרשה חריגה מהנרתיק?
Are you a high-risk pregnancy?	✖	✔	האם את בהריון בסיכון גבוה?
Have you had a recent physical injury?	✖	✔	האם הייתה לך פציעה גופנית לאחרונה?
Have you had complications with a past pregnancy?	✖	✔	האם היו לך סיבוכים בהריון קודם?

צייני כמה שבועות עברו מאז המחזור החודשי האחרון שלך.
Indicate how many weeks have passed since your last menstrual period.

<   1   2   3   4   5   6   7   8   9

צייני כמה חודשים את בהריון.
Indicate how many months you have been pregnant.

<   1   2   3   4   5   6   7   8   9

צייני את תאריך הלידה הצפוי.
Indicate what date you are due to give birth.

1 2 3 4 5 6 7			
8 9 10 11 12 13 14	ספטמבר September	מאי May	ינואר January
15 16 17 18 19 20 21	אוקטובר October	יוני June	פברואר February
22 23 24 25 26 27 28	נובמבר November	יולי July	מרץ March
29 30 31	דצמבר December	אוגוסט August	אפריל April

צייני כמה פעמים היית בהריון.
Indicate how many times you have been pregnant.

0   1   2   3   4   5   6   7   8   9

צייני כמה ילדים יש לך.
Indicate how many children you have.

0   1   2   3   4   5   6   7   8   9

צייני כמה הפלות מלאכותיות או הפלות טבעיות עברת.
Indicate how many abortions or miscarriages you have had.

0   1   2   3   4   5   6   7   8   9

תוך זמן קצר י/תהיה כאן מתורגמן/ית.
An interpreter will be here shortly.

נא לתת שתן בכלי זה. לאחר מכן, נא לסגור את המכסה ולתת לי את הכלי.
Please urinate in this cup. When you are finished, please attach the lid.

אני צריך/ה להכניס עירוי לווריד. זה עלול להכאיב במקצת.
I need to start an IV. This may hurt a little.

אני צריך/ה להניח מספר מדבקות על החזה שלך כדי לבדוק את הלב שלך.
I need to put some stickers on your chest in order to examine your heart.

אני צריך/ה להכניס צינורית לשלפוחית השתן שלך. זה יגרום לך לאי נוחות.
I need to put a tube in your bladder. This will be uncomfortable.

אני צריך/ה לבדוק את הראש והפנים שלך.
I need to examine your head and face.

נא לפתוח את הפה.
Please open your mouth.

אני צריך/ה לבדוק את החזה, הלב והריאות שלך.
I need to examine your chest, heart, and lungs.

אני צריך/ה לבדוק את הבטן שלך. זה עלול לגרום לך לאי נוחות.
I need to examine your abdomen. Slight discomfort may occur.

אני צריך/ה לבדוק את האגן ופי הטבעת שלך. זה עלול לגרום לך לאי נוחות.
I need to examine your pelvis and rectum. Slight discomfort may occur.

אני עומד/ת לתת לך תרופה שעלולה לגרום לך לאי נוחות זמנית.
I am going to give you a medication that may cause temporary discomfort.

אני עומד/ת לתת לך תרופה שיכולה לגרום לך לחוש נמנום או סחרחורת באופן זמני.
I am going to give you a medication that may make you feel sleepy or light-headed.

אני עומד/ת לקחת אותך לעבור סריקה רפואית. זה לא יכאב.
I am going to take you to get a medical scan. This will not hurt.

हैलो, मैं एक स्वास्थ्य देखभाल पेशेवर हूँ। मैं हिन्दी नहीं बोलता/बोलती हूँ।
Hello, I am a healthcare professional. I do not speak Hindi.

मुझे केवल हाँ या नहीं में जवाब दीजिये।
Respond to me only *yes* or *no*.

मुझे है ?
Do you have?

सर-दर्द	✔	✖	*A Headache*
चक्कर आते हैं	✔	✖	*Dizziness*
बुखार	✔	✖	*A Fever*
छाती में दर्द	✔	✖	*Chest Pain*
पूरी साँस लेने में तकलीफ	✔	✖	*SOB*
पेट में दर्द	✔	✖	*ABD Pain*
मितली होती है	✔	✖	*Nausea*
उल्टियाँ	✔	✖	*Vomiting*
अतिसार	✔	✖	*Diarrhea*
सूजन है	✔	✖	*Swelling*
नई कमजोरी है	✔	✖	*New Weakness*

हैलो, मैं एक स्वास्थ्य देखभाल पेशेवर हूँ। मैं हिन्दी नहीं बोलता/बोलती हूँ।

Hello, I am a healthcare professional. I do not speak Hindi.

कृपया (व्यक्ति के इस चित्र में) इशारा करके बताइये कि आपको कहाँ दर्द है।

Please point (on this picture of a person) to where you have pain.

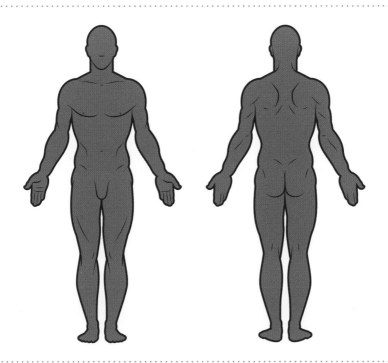

अपने दर्द का मूल्याँकन करने के लिए कृपया (इस स्केल पर) बिन्दु लगाएं।

Please point (on this scale) to rate your pain:

कोई दर्द नहीं	हल्का दर्द	भयंकर दर्द

0 1 2 3 4 5 6 7 8 9 10

मुझे केवल हाँ या नहीं में जवाब दीजिये।

Respond to me only yes or no.   *Do/Have you had:*

क्या आपको दवाएं लेने से एलर्जी है?	✓ ✗	*Rx Allergies*
क्या आपको अस्थमा है?	✓ ✗	*Asthma*
क्या आपका कैंसर का कोई इतिहास है?	✓ ✗	*Hx of Ca*
क्या आपको काँजेस्टिव ह्दय विफलता है?	✓ ✗	*CHF*
क्या आपका गुर्दे की विफलता का कोई इतिहास है?	✓ ✗	*CRF*
क्या आपको कभी पक्षाघात हुआ है?	✓ ✗	*CVA*
क्या आपको मधुमेह है?	✓ ✗	*DM*
क्या आपको वातस्फीति है?	✓ ✗	*Emphysema*
क्या आपको एच.आई.वी. या एड्स है?	✓ ✗	*HIV/AIDS*
क्या आपको उच्च रक्तचाप है?	✓ ✗	*HTN*
क्या आपको कभी दिल का दौरा पड़ा है?	✓ ✗	*An MI*
क्या आपको कोई मनोवैज्ञानिक समस्याएं हैं?	✓ ✗	*Psych Issues*
क्या अभी हाल ही आपकी कोई शल्यक्रिया हुई है?	✓ ✗	*Recent Surgery*
क्या आपका सीजर्स का कोई इतिहास है?	✓ ✗	*Hx of Sz*

HINDI / हिन्दी

52

हैलो, मैं एक स्वास्थ्य देखभाल पेशेवर हूँ। मैं हिन्दी नहीं बोलता/बोलती हूँ।
Hello, I am a healthcare professional. I do not speak Hindi.

मुझे केवल हाँ या नहीं में जवाब दीजिये।
Respond to me only *yes* or *no*.

क्या आप गर्भवती हैं?	✓	✗	Are you pregnant?
क्या आपको जलस्राव हुआ है?	✓	✗	Has your water broken?
क्या आपको संकुचन हो रहे हैं?	✓	✗	Are you having contractions?
क्या अब बच्चा बाहर आ रहा है?	✓	✗	Is the baby coming now?
क्या आपको पेट में दर्द है?	✓	✗	Do you have ABD pain?
क्या आपको योनि में दर्द है?	✓	✗	Do you have vaginal pain?
क्या आपको योनि से रक्तस्राव हो रहा है?	✓	✗	Do you have vaginal bleeding?
क्या आपकी योनि से असामान्य स्राव हो रहा है?	✓	✗	Do you have uncommon vaginal discharge?
क्या आपको उच्च जोखिम वाली गर्भावस्था है?	✓	✗	Are you a high-risk pregnancy?
क्या आपको अभी हाल ही में कोई शारीरिक चोट लगी है?	✓	✗	Have you had a recent physical injury?
क्या आपको पिछली गर्भावस्था के दौरान कोई जटिलता हुई थी?	✓	✗	Have you had complications with a past pregnancy?

बताइये कि आपके पिछले मासिक चक्र के पश्चात कितने सप्ताह गुजर चुके हैं।
Indicate how many weeks have passed since your last menstrual period.

<   1   2   3   4   5   6   7   8   9

बताइये कि आप कितने महीने की गर्भवती हैं।
Indicate how many months you have been pregnant.

<   1   2   3   4   5   6   7   8   9

उस तिथि को इंगित करें जब आपकी बच्चे को जन्म देने की संभावना है?
Indicate what date you are due to give birth.

जनवरी January	मई May	सितंबर September	1	2	3	4	5	6	7
फरवरी February	जून June	अक्टूबर October	8	9	10	11	12	13	14
			15	16	17	18	19	20	21
मार्च March	जुलाई July	नवंबर November	22	23	24	25	26	27	28
अप्रैल April	अगस्त August	दिसंबर December	29	30	31				

बताइये कि आप कितनी बार गर्भवती हो चुकी हैं।
Indicate how many times you have been pregnant.

0   1   2   3   4   5   6   7   8   9

बताइये कि आपके कितने बच्चे हैं।
Indicate how many children you have.

0   1   2   3   4   5   6   7   8   9

बताइये कि आपको कितनी बार गर्भपात हो चुका है।
Indicate how many abortions or miscarriages you have had.

0   1   2   3   4   5   6   7   8   9

थोड़ी ही देर में यहाँ एक अनुवादक आएगा।
An interpreter will be here shortly.

कृपया इस कप में पेशाब करें। जब आप कर चुकें तो ढक्कन से ढंक दें।
Please urinate in this cup. When you are finished, please attach the lid.

मुझे आई.वी. आरंभ करना होगा। इससे थोड़ी तकलीफ होगी।
I need to start an IV. This may hurt a little.

मुझे आपके दिल की जाँच करने के लिए आपकी छाती पर कुछ स्टिकर लगाने होंगे।
I need to put some stickers on your chest in order to examine your heart.

मुझे आपके ब्लैडर में एक ट्यूब को डालना है। इससे परेशानी होगी।
I need to put a tube in your bladder. This will be uncomfortable.

मुझे आपके सिर और चेहरे का परीक्षण करना है।
I need to examine your head and face.

कृपया अपना मुँह खोलें।
Please open your mouth.

मुझे आपकी छाती, दिल और फेफड़ों की जाँच करनी है।
I need to examine your chest, heart, and lungs.

मुझे आपके पेट की जाँच करनी है। इससे परेशानी हो सकती है।
I need to examine your abdomen. Slight discomfort may occur.

मुझे आपकी श्रोणि और गुदा की जाँच करनी है। इससे परेशानी हो सकती है।
I need to examine your pelvis and rectum. Slight discomfort may occur.

मैं आपको दवा देने जा रहा/ रही हूँ जिससे आपको अस्थाई रूप से परेशानी हो सकती है।
I am going to give you a medication that may cause temporary discomfort.

मैं आपको दवा देने जा रहा/ रही हूँ जिससे आपको अस्थाई रूप से उनींदापन या चंचलता महसूस हो सकती है।
I am going to give you a medication that may make you feel sleepy or light-headed.

मैं आपको आपके चिकित्सीय स्कैन के लिए ले जा रहा/रही हूँ। इससे तकलीफ नहीं होगी।
I am going to take you to get a medical scan. This will not hurt.

Salve, sono un professionista sanitario. Non parlo Italiano.

Hello, I am a healthcare professional. I do not speak Italian

Mi risponda solo sì o no.

Respond to me only *yes* or *no*.

Quali sono i suoi sintomi?

Do you have?

Italiano	Sì	No	English
Mal di testa	✓	✗	*A Headache*
Capogiri	✓	✗	*Dizziness*
Febbre	✓	✗	*A Fever*
Dolore al torace	✓	✗	*Chest Pain*
Respiro affannoso	✓	✗	*SOB*
Dolore addominale	✓	✗	*ABD Pain*
Nausea	✓	✗	*Nausea*
Vomito	✓	✗	*Vomiting*
Diarrea	✓	✗	*Diarrhea*
Gonfiore	✓	✗	*Swelling*
Debolezza recente	✓	✗	*New Weakness*

Salve, sono un professionista sanitario. Non parlo Italiano.

Hello, I am a healthcare professional. I do not speak Italian.

Indichi (su quest'immagine di una persona) dove sente dolore.

Please point (on this picture of a person) to where you have pain.

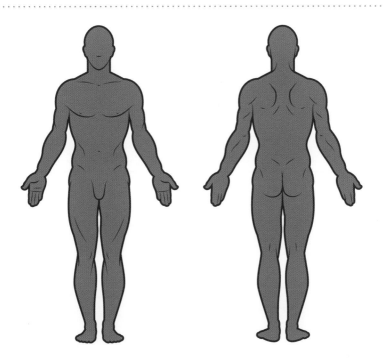

Indichi (su questa scala) l'intensità del dolore che avverte.

Please point (on this scale) to rate your pain:

Nessun dolore   Dolore moderato   Dolore intenso

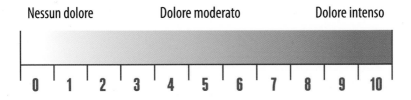

0   1   2   3   4   5   6   7   8   9   10

Mi risponda solo sì o no.
Respond to me only *yes* or *no*.

Do/Have you had:

È allergico/a a qualche medicamento?	✓	✗	Rx Allergies
Soffre di asma?	✓	✗	Asthma
Ha mai avuto il cancro?	✓	✗	Hx of Ca
Soffre di insufficienza cardiaca congestizia?	✓	✗	CHF
Ha mai sofferto di insufficienza renale?	✓	✗	CRF
Ha mai avuto un ictus?	✓	✗	CVA
È diabetico/a?	✓	✗	DM
Soffre di enfisema?	✓	✗	Emphysema
È sieropositivo/a per l'HIV o ha l'AIDS?	✓	✗	HIV/AIDS
Ha la pressione alta?	✓	✗	HTN
Ha mai avuto un attacco cardiaco?	✓	✗	An MI
Soffre di problemi psicologici?	✓	✗	Psych Issues
Si è sottoposto/a recentemente a un intervento chirurgico?	✓	✗	Recent Surgery
Soffre o ha sofferto di convulsioni?	✓	✗	Hx of Sz

ITALIAN / ITALIANO

58

Salve, sono un professionista sanitario. Non parlo Italiano.
Hello, I am a healthcare professional. I do not speak Italian.

Mi risponda solo sì o no.
Respond to me only *yes* or *no*.

È incinta?	✓	✗	*Are you pregnant?*
Le si sono rotte le acque?	✓	✗	*Has your water broken?*
Sta avendo le contrazioni?	✓	✗	*Are you having contractions?*
Il bambino sta nascendo adesso?	✓	✗	*Is the baby coming now?*
Sente dolore addominale?	✓	✗	*Do you have ABD pain?*
Sente dolore vaginale?	✓	✗	*Do you have vaginal pain?*
Sente un'emorragia vaginale?	✓	✗	*Do you have vaginal bleeding?*
Ha perdite insolite dalla vagina?	✓	✗	*Do you have uncommon vaginal discharge?*
La sua è una gravidanza ad alto rischio?	✓	✗	*Are you a high-risk pregnancy?*
Di recente ha subito lesioni fisiche?	✓	✗	*Have you had a recent physical injury?*
Ha avuto complicazioni in una gravidanza precedente?	✓	✗	*Have you had complications with a past pregnancy?*

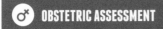
Indichi quante settimane sono trascorse dal suo ultimo periodo mestruale.

Indicate how many weeks have passed since your last menstrual period.

<   1   2   3   4   5   6   7   8   9

Indichi da quanti mesi è incinta.

Indicate how many months you have been pregnant.

<   1   2   3   4   5   6   7   8   9

Indichi la data prevista per il parto.

Indicate what date you are due to give birth.

Gennaio January	Maggio May	Settembre September	1 2 3 4 5 6 7
Febbraio February	Giugno June	Ottobre October	8 9 10 11 12 13 14
			15 16 17 18 19 20 21
Marzo March	Luglio July	Novembre November	22 23 24 25 26 27 28
Aprile April	Agosto August	Dicembre December	29 30 31

Indichi quante gravidanze ha avuto.

Indicate how many times you have been pregnant.

0   1   2   3   4   5   6   7   8   9

Indichi quanti figli ha.

Indicate how many children you have.

0   1   2   3   4   5   6   7   8   9

Indichi quanti aborti o aborti spontanei ha avuto.

Indicate how many abortions or miscarriages you have had.

0   1   2   3   4   5   6   7   8   9

Un interprete arriverà tra poco.
An interpreter will be here shortly.

Urini in questo contenitore. Quando ha finito, lo chiuda con il coperchio e me lo dia.
Please urinate in this cup. When you are finished, please attach the lid.

Devo farle una flebo. Potrebbe sentire un po' di dolore.
I need to start an IV. This may hurt a little.

Devo applicarle degli elettrodi adesivi sul torace per esaminarle il cuore.
I need to put some stickers on your chest in order to examine your heart.

Devo inserirle un catetere nella vescica. Questo le darà fastidio.
I need to put a tube in your bladder. This will be uncomfortable.

Devo esaminarle la testa e il viso.
I need to examine your head and face.

Apra la bocca.
Please open your mouth.

Devo esaminarle il torace, il cuore e i polmoni.
I need to examine your chest, heart, and lungs.

Devo esaminarle l'addome. Potrebbe sentire un certo fastidio
I need to examine your abdomen. Slight discomfort may occur.

Devo esaminarle il bacino e il retto. Potrebbe sentire un certo fastidio.
I need to examine your pelvis and rectum. Slight discomfort may occur.

Le somministrerò un medicamento che potrà darle temporaneamente fastidio.
I am going to give you a medication that may cause temporary discomfort.

Le somministrerò un medicamento che potrebbe farla sentire temporaneamente sonnolenta o con il capogiro.
I am going to give you a medication that may make you feel sleepy or light-headed.

La porterò a fare un' ecografia. Non sentirà alcun dolore.
I am going to take you to get a medical scan. This will not hurt.

こんにちは。私はヘルスケアの専門家です。でも日本語は話せません。
Hello, I am a healthcare professional. I do not speak Japanese.

私の質問に、「はい」か「いいえ」で答えてください。
Respond to me only *yes* or *no*.

次のような症状がありますか？
Do you have?

頭痛	✓	✗	*A Headache*
めまい	✓	✗	*Dizziness*
熱	✓	✗	*A Fever*
胸の痛み	✓	✗	*Chest Pain*
息切れ	✓	✗	*SOB*
腹痛	✓	✗	*ABD Pain*
吐き気	✓	✗	*Nausea*
嘔吐	✓	✗	*Vomiting*
下痢	✓	✗	*Diarrhea*
腫れ・むくみ	✓	✗	*Swelling*
倦怠感	✓	✗	*New Weakness*

JAPANESE / 日本語

62

こんにちは。私はヘルスケアの専門家です。でも日本語は話せません。
Hello, I am a healthcare professional. I do not speak Japanese.

（人体図上で）痛いところを 指差してください。
Please point (on this picture of a person) to where you have pain.

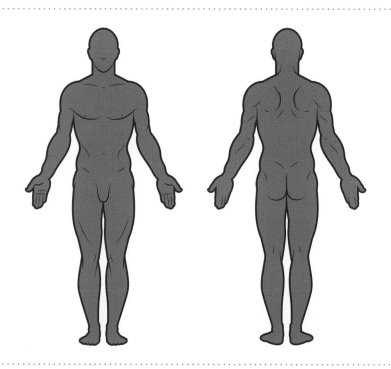

痛みの程度について、指差してください。
Please point (on this scale) to rate your pain:

痛みはない　　　　少し痛む　　　　ひどく痛む

| 0 | 1 | 2 | 3 | 4 | 5 | 6 | 7 | 8 | 9 | 10 |

JAPANESE / 日本語

私の質問に、「はい」か「いいえ」で答えてください。

Respond to me only *yes* or *no*.

Do/Have you had:

今までに服用してアレルギー反応を起こした薬はありますか?			*Rx Allergies*
喘息の症状がありますか?			*Asthma*
癌にかかったことがありますか?			*Hx of Ca*
うっ血性心不全にかかっていますか?			*CHF*
腎臓の機能不全になったことがありますか?			*CRF*
脳卒中になったことがありますか?			*CVA*
糖尿病にかかっていますか?			*DM*
肺気腫にかかっていますか?			*Emphysema*
HIVまたはエイズにかかっていますか?			*HIV/AIDS*
高血圧ですか?			*HTN*
心臓発作を起こしたことがありますか?			*An MI*
うつやパニック症候群など精神的な問題を抱えていますか?			*Psych Issues*
最近手術をしましたか?			*Recent Surgery*
発作が起きたことはありますか?			*Hx of Sz*

JAPANESE / 日本語

64

こんにちは。私はヘルスケアの専門家です。でも日本語は話せません。
Hello, I am a healthcare professional. I do not speak Japanese.

私の質問に、「はい」か「いいえ」で答えてください。
Respond to me only *yes* or *no*.

妊娠していますか？   *Are you pregnant?*

破水しましたか？   *Has your water broken?*

子宮の収縮が始まりましたか？   *Are you having contractions?*

すでに赤ちゃんが下がってきていますか？   *Is the baby coming now?*

腹部に痛みはありますか？   *Do you have ABD pain?*

膣内に痛みはありますか？   *Do you have vaginal pain?*

膣内出血がありますか？   *Do you have vaginal bleeding?*

普段と異なる膣内分泌物がありますか？   *Do you have uncommon vaginal discharge?*

子宮外妊娠などリスクの高い妊娠状態ですか？   *Are you a high-risk pregnancy?*

最近身体のどこかを怪我しましたか？   *Have you had a recent physical injury?*

過去の妊娠で合併症を起こしたことはありますか？   *Have you had complications with a past pregnancy?*

最後に生理があったのは何週間前ですか。
Indicate how many weeks have passed since your last menstrual period.

< 1 2 3 4 5 6 7 8 9

現在妊娠何カ月ですか。
Indicate how many months you have been pregnant.

< 1 2 3 4 5 6 7 8 9

出産予定日を教えてください。
Indicate what date you are due to give birth.

1月 January	5月 May	9月 September	1 2 3 4 5 6 7
2月 February	6月 June	10月 October	8 9 10 11 12 13 14
3月 March	7月 July	11月 November	15 16 17 18 19 20 21
4月 April	8月 August	12月 December	22 23 24 25 26 27 28
			29 30 31

今までに何度妊娠したことがありますか。
Indicate how many times you have been pregnant.

0 1 2 3 4 5 6 7 8 9

子供は何人いますか。
Indicate how many children you have.

0 1 2 3 4 5 6 7 8 9

今までに中絶または流産したことがありますか。それは何度ありますか。
Indicate how many abortions or miscarriages you have had.

0 1 2 3 4 5 6 7 8 9

通訳がもうすぐ到着します。
An interpreter will be here shortly.

このカップに尿を入れてきてください。
終わったらフタをして、カップを持って戻ってきてください。そして私に渡してください。
Please urinate in this cup. When you are finished, please attach the lid.

点滴を始める必要があります。少し痛いですが我慢してください。
I need to start an IV. This may hurt a little.

心臓の検査をしますので、今から胸にシールを貼ります。
I need to put some stickers on your chest in order to examine your heart.

膀胱に管を通す必要があります。少し気持ち悪いかも知れません。
I need to put a tube in your bladder. This will be uncomfortable.

頭と顔をチェックする必要があります。
I need to examine your head and face.

口を開けてください。
Please open your mouth.

胸と心臓、および肺をチェックする必要があります。
I need to examine your chest, heart, and lungs.

腹部をチェックする必要があります。少し気持ち悪いかも知れません。
I need to examine your abdomen. Slight discomfort may occur.

骨盤と腸をチェックする必要があります。少し気持ち悪いかも知れません。
I need to examine your pelvis and rectum. Slight discomfort may occur.

今から渡す薬を飲むと少し不快な気分になるかも知れませんが、しばらくの間だけです。
I am going to give you a medication that may cause temporary discomfort.

今から渡す薬を飲むと眠くなったり頭がぼーっとするかも知れませんが、しばらくの間だけです。
I am going to give you a medication that may make you feel sleepy or light-headed.

今からあなたの身体をスキャンする検査室へ行きます。これは痛くないので心配する必要はありません。
I am going to take you to get a medical scan. This will not hurt.

안녕하세요. 저는 의료 전문가입니다. 저는 한국어를 못합니다.
Hello, I am a healthcare professional. I do not speak Korean.

네 혹은 아니오라고만 대답해 주십시오.
Respond to me only *yes* or *no*.

아래의 증상이 있으십니까?
Do you have?

두통	✓	✗	*A Headache*
현기증	✓	✗	*Dizziness*
열	✓	✗	*A Fever*
가슴이 아픔	✓	✗	*Chest Pain*
숨이 가쁨	✓	✗	*SOB*
복통	✓	✗	*ABD Pain*
메스꺼움	✓	✗	*Nausea*
토했음	✓	✗	*Vomiting*
설사	✓	✗	*Diarrhea*
부기	✓	✗	*Swelling*
새로운 쇠약	✓	✗	*New Weakness*

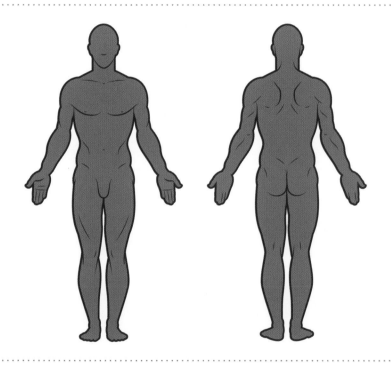

KOREAN / 한국어

68

안녕하세요. 저는 의료 전문가입니다. 저는 한국어를 못합니다.
Hello, I am a healthcare professional. I do not speak Korean.

(이 사람 그림에서) 통증이 있는 부위를 손으로가리켜 보세요.
Please point (on this picture of a person) to where you have pain.

(아래의 척도에서) 통증을 평가하기 위해 손가락으로 가리키십시오.
Please point (on this scale) to rate your pain.

무통증	보통의 통증	심한 통증

0	1	2	3	4	5	6	7	8	9	10

네 혹은 아니오라고만 대답해 주십시오.
Respond to me only *yes* or *no*.   *Do/Have you had:*

약에 알레르기가 있으십니까?   *Rx Allergies*

천식이 있으십니까?   *Asthma*

암에 걸리신 적이 있으십니까?   *Hx of Ca*

울혈성 심부전이 있으십니까?   *CHF*

신부전이 있으신 적이 있으십니까?   *CRF*

뇌졸중이 있으신 적이 있으십니까?   *CVA*

당뇨병이 있으십니까?   *DM*

폐기종이 있으십니까?   *Emphysema*

HIV나 에이즈가 있으십니까?   *HIV/AIDS*

고혈압이 있으십니까?   *HTN*

심장 마비 증상이 있으십니까?   *An MI*

심리적 문제가 있습니까?   *Psych Issues*

최근에 수술하셨습니까?   *Recent Surgery*

간질 발작이 있으신 적이 있습니까?   *Hx of Sz*

KOREAN / 한국어

70

안녕하세요. 저는 의료 전문가입니다. 저는 한국어를 못합니다.
Hello, I am a healthcare professional. I do not speak Korean.

네 혹은 아니오라고만 대답해 주십시오.
Respond to me only *yes* or *no*.

Korean	✓	✗	English
임신하셨습니까?	✓	✗	Are you pregnant?
양수가 터졌습니까?	✓	✗	Has your water broken?
진통이 있으십니까?	✓	✗	Are you having contractions?
지금 아기가 나오고 있습니까?	✓	✗	Is the baby coming now?
복통이 있으십니까?	✓	✗	Do you have ABD pain?
질 통증이 있으십니까?	✓	✗	Do you have vaginal pain?
질 출혈이 있으십니까?	✓	✗	Do you have vaginal bleeding?
흔치 않은 질 분비물이 있으십니까?	✓	✗	Do you have uncommon vaginal discharge?
고위험 임신이십니까?	✓	✗	Are you a high-risk pregnancy?
최근에 육체적 상해를 입으셨습니까?	✓	✗	Have you had a recent physical injury?
과거 임신에서 합병증이 있었습니까?	✓	✗	Have you had complications with a past pregnancy?

마지막 월경이 있고 몇 주나 지났는지 알려 주세요.
Indicate how many weeks have passed since your last menstrual period.

<   1   2   3   4   5   6   7   8   9

임신한 지 몇 달이 되었는지 알려 주세요.
Indicate how many months you have been pregnant.

<   1   2   3   4   5   6   7   8   9

임신 예정일을 알려주십시오.
Indicate what date you are due to give birth.

1월 January	5월 May	9월 September	1 2 3 4 5 6 7
2월 February	6월 June	10월 October	8 9 10 11 12 13 14
3월 March	7월 July	11월 November	15 16 17 18 19 20 21 22 23 24 25 26 27 28
4월 April	8월 August	12월 December	29 30 31

몇 번이나 임신했는지 알려 주세요.
Indicate how many times you have been pregnant.

0   1   2   3   4   5   6   7   8   9

자녀가 몇이나 되는지 알려 주세요.
Indicate how many children you have.

0   1   2   3   4   5   6   7   8   9

낙태 혹은 유산을 몇 번이나 했는지 알려주세요.
Indicate how many abortions or miscarriages you have had.

0   1   2   3   4   5   6   7   8   9

통역사가 곧 올 겁니다.
An interpreter will be here shortly.

이 컵에 소변을 보아주십시오. 소변을 보셨으면 뚜껑을 덮어서 컵을 제게 주십시오.
Please urinate in this cup. When you are finished, please attach the lid.

정맥주사를 시작해야 합니다. 좀 아프실 수 있습니다.
I need to start an IV. This may hurt a little.

심장을 검진하기 위해서 가슴에 스티커들을 붙여야 합니다.
I need to put some stickers on your chest in order to examine your heart.

방광에 튜브를 넣어야 합니다. 불편하실 겁니다.
I need to put a tube in your bladder. This will be uncomfortable.

머리와 얼굴을 검진해야 합니다.
I need to examine your head and face.

입을 벌려주십시오.
Please open your mouth.

가슴, 심장, 및 허파를 검진해야 합니다.
I need to examine your chest, heart, and lungs.

복부를 검진해야 합니다. 불편하실 수 있습니다.
I need to examine your abdomen. Slight discomfort may occur.

골반과 직장을 검진해야 합니다. 불편하실 수 있습니다.
I need to examine your pelvis and rectum. Slight discomfort may occur.

일어나셔서 잠깐 걸어 주십시오.
I am going to give you a medication that may cause temporary discomfort.

제가 약을 드리겠는데 잠시 졸리거나 어지러울 수 있습니다.
I am going to give you a medication that may make you feel sleepy or light-headed.

의료 촬영을 위해 모시고 가겠습니다. 아프지 않을 겁니다.
I am going to take you to get a medical scan. This will not hurt.

سلام، من متخصص مراقبت‌های بهداشتی هستم. من به زبان فارسی صحبت نمی‌کنم.

Hello, I am a healthcare professional. I do not speak Persian.

به من فقط با بله یا خیر پاسخ دهید.

Respond to me only *yes* or *no*.

آیا شما دارای یکی از این بیماری‌ها یا ناراحتی‌های زیر هستید؟

Do you have?

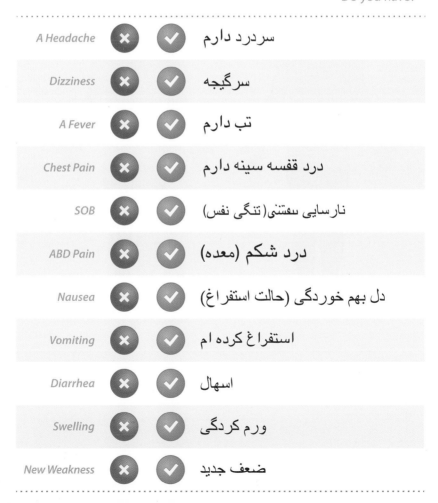

A Headache	✖	✔	سردرد دارم
Dizziness	✖	✔	سرگیجه
A Fever	✖	✔	تب دارم
Chest Pain	✖	✔	درد قفسه سینه دارم
SOB	✖	✔	نارسایی سفتنی (تنگی نفس)
ABD Pain	✖	✔	درد شکم (معده)
Nausea	✖	✔	دل بهم خوردگی (حالت استفراغ)
Vomiting	✖	✔	استفراغ کرده ام
Diarrhea	✖	✔	اسهال
Swelling	✖	✔	ورم کردگی
New Weakness	✖	✔	ضعف جدید

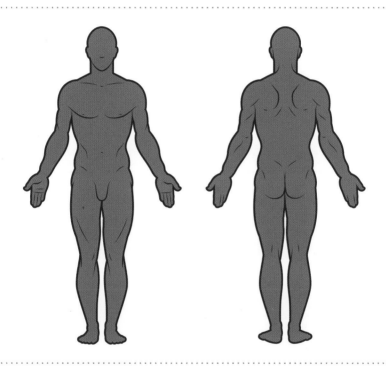

PERSIAN / فارسی

سلام، من متخصص مراقبت‌های بهداشتی هستم. من به زبان فارسی صحبت نمی‌کنم.

Hello, I am a healthcare professional. I do not speak Persian.

لطفا، با اشاره (بر روی عکس) مشخص کنید که درد در کدام قسمت بدنتان می‌باشد.

Please point (on this picture of a person) to where you have pain.

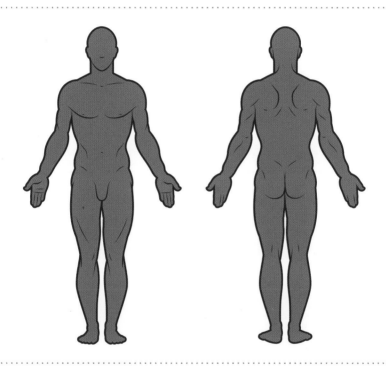

لطفا، با اشاره (بر روی این مقیاس) میزان درد خود را مشخص کنید.

Please point (on this scale) to rate your pain:

دردی وجود ندارد   درد متوسط   درد شدید

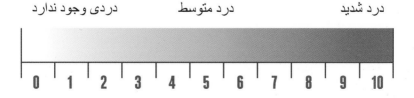

0   1   2   3   4   5   6   7   8   9   10

Do/Have you had:

به من فقط با بله یا خیر پاسخ دهید.

Respond to me only *yes* or *no*.

Rx Allergies	✖	✔	آیا حساسیت دارویی داری؟
Asthma	✖	✔	آیا بیماری آسم داشته‌اید؟
Hx of Ca	✖	✔	ایا آسابقه بیماری سرطان داشته‌اید؟
CHF	✖	✔	آیا سابقه نارسایی احتقانی قلبی داشته‌اید؟
CRF	✖	✔	آیا سابقه وقفه کلیه داشته‌اید؟
CVA	✖	✔	آیا سابقه سکته قلبی داشته‌اید؟
DM	✖	✔	آیا بیماری قند (دیابت) دارید؟
Emphysema	✖	✔	آمفیزم (امفسیما) دارید؟
HIV/AIDS	✖	✔	آیا اچ-آی-وی یا بیماری ایدز دارید؟
HTN	✖	✔	آیا فشار خون بالا دارید؟
An MI	✖	✔	آیا حمله قلبی داشته اید؟
Psych Issues	✖	✔	آیا مشکلات روانی دارید؟
Recent Surgery	✖	✔	آیا اخیراً جراحی داشته‌اید؟
Hx of Sz	✖	✔	آیا سابقه بیماری صرع داشته‌اید؟

PERSIAN / فارسی

76

سلام, من متخصص مراقبت‌های بهداشتی هستم. من به زبان فارسی صحبت نمی‌کنم.
Hello, I am a healthcare professional. I do not speak Persian.

به من فقط با بله یا خیر پاسخ دهید.
Respond to me only *yes* or *no*.

Are you pregnant?	✖	✔	آیا حامله هستید؟
Has your water broken?	✖	✔	آیا کیسه آب شما پاره شده است؟
Are you having contractions?	✖	✔	آیا دارای انقباضات ماهیچه‌ای هستید؟
Is the baby coming now?	✖	✔	آیا کودک در حال به دنیا آمدن است؟
Do you have ABD pain?	✖	✔	آیا درد شکم دارید؟
Do you have vaginal pain?	✖	✔	آیا درد مهبل (واژن) دارید؟
Do you have vaginal bleeding?	✖	✔	آیا خون‌ریزی مهبلی (مهبلی) دارید؟
Do you have uncommon vaginal discharge?	✖	✔	آیا ترشح غیرعادی از مهبل (واژن) دارید؟
Are you a high-risk pregnancy?	✖	✔	آیا حاملگی برای شما خطر زیادی دارد؟
Have you had a recent physical injury?	✖	✔	آیا اخیراً صدمه بدنی داشته‌اید؟
Have you had complications with a past pregnancy?	✖	✔	آیا در حاملگی‌های گذشته مشکلاتی داشته؟

مشخص کنید چند هفته از آخرین قاعدگیتان گذشته است؟

Indicate how many weeks have passed since your last menstrual period.

<   1   2   3   4   5   6   7   8   9

مشخص کنید چند ماهه حامله هستید؟

Indicate how many months you have been pregnant.

<   1   2   3   4   5   6   7   8   9

تاریخی را که موعد زایمانتان است، نشان بدهید.

Indicate what date you are due to give birth.

1	2	3	4	5	6	7	سپتامبر September	می May	ژانویه January
8	9	10	11	12	13	14	اوکتبر October	جون June	فوریه February
15	16	17	18	19	20	21	نوامبر November	جولای July	مارچ March
22	23	24	25	26	27	28	دسامبر December	اوگوست August	آوریل April
29	30	31							

نشان بدهید چند بار حامله شده‌اید.

Indicate how many times you have been pregnant.

0   1   2   3   4   5   6   7   8   9

نشان بدهید چند تا فرزند دارید.

Indicate how many children you have.

0   1   2   3   4   5   6   7   8   9

نشان بدهید چند بار سقط جنین (کورتاژ) یا سقط جنین خود به خوداشته‌اید.

Indicate how many abortions or miscarriages you have had.

0   1   2   3   4   5   6   7   8   9

بزودی مترجمی اینجا خواهد آمد.

An interpreter will be here shortly.

لطفاً در این لیوان ادرار کنید. وقتی که تمام کردید، لطفاً در آن را بگذارید و به من بدهید.

Please urinate in this cup. When you are finished, please attach the lid.

من باید تزریق سرم را شروع کنم. این عمل ممکن است کمی درد داشته باشد.

I need to start an IV. This may hurt a little.

من برای معاینه قلبتان باید تعدادی وصله بر روی سینه شما بگذارم.

I need to put some stickers on your chest in order to examine your heart.

من بایدلوله‌ای را وارد مثانه شما بکنم. این عمل کمی ناراحتی ایجاد می‌کند.

I need to put a tube in your bladder. This will be uncomfortable.

من باید سر و صورت شما را معاینه کنم.

I need to examine your head and face.

لطفاً دهانتان را باز کنید.

Please open your mouth.

من باید سینه، قلب و شش‌های شما را معاینه کنم.

I need to examine your chest, heart, and lungs.

من باید شکمتان را معاینه کنم. این ممکن است ناراحتی ایجاد کند.

I need to examine your abdomen. Slight discomfort may occur.

من باید لگن و راست روده (قسمت انتهائی روده بزرگ) شما را معاینه کنم.

I need to examine your pelvis and rectum. Slight discomfort may occur.

من به شما داروئی می‌دهم که ممکن است بطور موقت برای شما ناراحتی ایجاد کند.

I am going to give you a medication that may cause temporary discomfort.

من به شما داروئی را می‌دهم که ممکن است برای شمابطور موقت خواب آلودگی ایجاد کند.

I am going to give you a medication that may make you feel sleepy or light-headed.

من شما را برای یک عکس‌برداری پزشکی می‌برم. این عمل دردی ندارد.

I am going to take you to get a medical scan. This will not hurt.

Dzień dobry, jestem pracownikiem służby zdrowia. Nie mówię po polsku.
Hello, I am a healthcare professional. I do not speak Polish.

Proszę odpowiadać na moje pytania TAK lub NIE.
Respond to me only *yes* or *no*.

Czy masz któreś z poniższych objawów?
Do you have?

Ból głowy	✓	✗	*A Headache*
Zawroty głowy	✓	✗	*Dizziness*
Gorączka	✓	✗	*A Fever*
Ból w klatce piersiowej	✓	✗	*Chest Pain*
Zadyszka, duszności	✓	✗	*SOB*
Bóle brzucha	✓	✗	*ABD Pain*
Mdłości	✓	✗	*Nausea*
Wymioty	✓	✗	*Vomiting*
Biegunka	✓	✗	*Diarrhea*
Opuchlizna, obrzęki	✓	✗	*Swelling*
Osłabienie, które występuje od niedawna	✓	✗	*New Weakness*

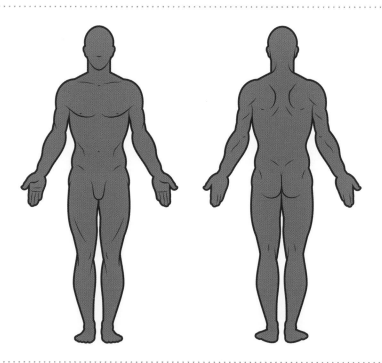

POLISH / Polski

Dzień dobry, jestem pracownikiem służby zdrowia. Nie mówię po polsku.
Hello, I am a healthcare professional. I do not speak Polish.

Wskaż na rysunku, gdzie odczuwasz ból.
Please point (on this picture of a person) to where you have pain.

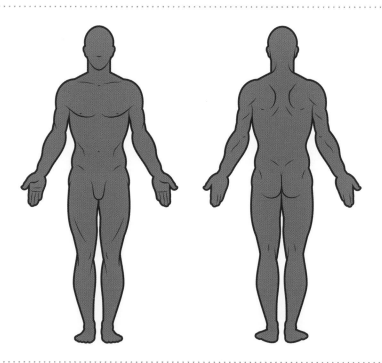

Wskaż na poniższej skali, jak bardzo Cię boli.
Please point (on this scale) to rate your pain.

Nic mnie nie boli	Umiarkowany ból	Silny ból

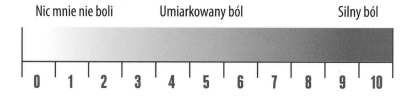

0 1 2 3 4 5 6 7 8 9 10

Proszę odpowiadać na moje pytania TAK lub NIE.
Respond to me only *yes* or *no*.

Do/Have you had:

Czy masz uczulenie na jakieś leki? ✓ ✗ *Rx Allergies*

Czy masz astmę? ✓ ✗ *Asthma*

Czy miałaś (miałeś) w przeszłości lub masz obecnie chorobę nowotworową? ✓ ✗ *Hx of Ca*

Czy cierpisz na zastoinową niewydolność serca? ✓ ✗ *CHF*

Czy miałaś (miałeś) lub masz ostrą niewydolność nerek albo osłabienie czynności nerek? ✓ ✗ *CRF*

Czy kiedykolwiek miałaś (miałeś) udar mózgu albo zawał mięśnia sercowego? ✓ ✗ *CVA*

Czy masz cukrzycę? ✓ ✗ *DM*

Czy masz rozedmę płuc? ✓ ✗ *Emphysema*

Czy rozpoznano u Ciebie wirusa HIV, czy zdiagnozowano u Ciebie chorobę AIDS? ✓ ✗ *HIV/AIDS*

Czy masz wysokie ciśnienie krwi? ✓ ✗ *HTN*

Czy miałaś (miałeś) w przeszłości atak serca? ✓ ✗ *An MI*

Czy masz jakiś problem psychologiczny? ✓ ✗ *Psych Issues*

Czy przechodziłeś (aś) ostatnio jakąś operacje? ✓ ✗ *Recent Surgery*

Czy kiedykolwiek miałeś (aś) atak padaczki? ✓ ✗ *Hx of Sz*

POLISH / Polski

82

Dzień dobry, jestem pracownikiem służby zdrowia. Nie mówię po polsku.
Hello, I am a healthcare professional. I do not speak Polish.

Proszę odpowiadać na moje pytania TAK lub NIE.
Respond to me only *yes* or *no*.

Czy jesteś w ciąży?	✔ ✘	Are you pregnant?
Czy odeszły Ci wody płodowe?	✔ ✘	Has your water broken?
Czy odczuwasz skurcze?	✔ ✘	Are you having contractions?
Czy czujesz, że zbliża się poród?	✔ ✘	Is the baby coming now?
Czy odczuwasz bóle brzucha?	✔ ✘	Do you have ABD pain?
Czy odczuwasz bóle w pochwie?	✔ ✘	Do you have vaginal pain?
Czy zaobserwowałaś krwistą wydzielinę z pochwy?	✔ ✘	Do you have vaginal bleeding?
Czy zauważyłaś jakąś nietypową wydzielinę z pochwy?	✔ ✘	Do you have uncommon vaginal discharge?
Czy Twoja ciąża jest ciążą podwyższonego ryzyka?	✔ ✘	Are you a high-risk pregnancy?
Czy doznałaś ostatnio jakichś obrażeń ciała?	✔ ✘	Have you had a recent physical injury?
Czy Twoja poprzednia ciąża była ciążą z powikłaniami?	✔ ✘	Have you had complications with a past pregnancy?

Ile tygodni minęło od Twojej ostatniej miesiączki?
Indicate how many weeks have passed since your last menstrual period.

< 1 2 3 4 5 6 7 8 9

W którym miesiącu ciąży jesteś?
Indicate how many months you have been pregnant.

< 1 2 3 4 5 6 7 8 9

Podaj przewidywaną datę porodu.
Indicate what date you are due to give birth.

Styczeń January	Maj May	Wrzesień September	1 2 3 4 5 6 7
Luty February	Czerwiec June	Październik October	8 9 10 11 12 13 14
Marzec March	Lipiec July	Listopad November	15 16 17 18 19 20 21
Kwiecień April	Sierpień August	Grudzień December	22 23 24 25 26 27 28
			29 30 31

Podaj, która to Twoja ciąża.
Indicate how many times you have been pregnant.

0 1 2 3 4 5 6 7 8 9

Podaj, ile masz dzieci.
Indicate how many children you have.

0 1 2 3 4 5 6 7 8 9

Podaj, ile razy przeszłaś aborcję lub poronienie.
Indicate how many abortions or miscarriages you have had.

0 1 2 3 4 5 6 7 8 9

Tłumacz wkrótce przybędzie.
An interpreter will be here shortly.

Umieść w tym pojemniku próbkę moczu, a następnie zakręć pokrywkę.
Please urinate in this cup. When you are finished, please attach the lid.

Musimy podłączyć Ci kroplówkę. To może być trochę bolesne.
I need to start an IV. This may hurt a little.

Musimy nakleić na Twojej klatce piersiowej plastry, by zbadać pracę Twojego serca.
I need to put some stickers on your chest in order to examine your heart.

Musimy wprowadzić cewnik do Twojego pęcherza moczowego. To dość nieprzyjemne.
I need to put a tube in your bladder. This will be uncomfortable.

Musimy zbadać Twoją głowę i twarz.
I need to examine your head and face.

Proszę otworzyć usta.
Please open your mouth.

Musimy zbadać Twoją klatkę piersiową, serce i płuca.
I need to examine your chest, heart, and lungs.

Musimy zbadać Twój brzuch. To może być nieco nieprzyjemne.
I need to examine your abdomen. Slight discomfort may occur.

Musimy zbadać Twoją miednicę i odbytnicę. To może być nieco nieprzyjemne.
I need to examine your pelvis and rectum. Slight discomfort may occur.

Teraz dostaniesz lekarstwo, które może spowodować chwilowo nieprzyjemne uczucie.
I am going to give you a medication that may cause temporary discomfort.

Teraz otrzymasz lek, który może spowodować chwilową senność lub oszołomienie.
I am going to give you a medication that may make you feel sleepy or light-headed.

Teraz zabierzemy Cię na dokładne badanie lekarskie. Badanie nie będzie bolesne.
I am going to take you to get a medical scan. This will not hurt.

Olá, eu sou um profissional da área de saúde. Eu não falo Português.
Hello, I am a healthcare professional. I do not speak Portuguese.

Responda minhas perguntas dizendo sim ou não.
Respond to me only *yes* or *no*.

Você tem?
Do you have?

Dor de cabeça	✓	✗	*A Headache*
Tontura	✓	✗	*Dizziness*
Febre	✓	✗	*A Fever*
Dores no peito	✓	✗	*Chest Pain*
Falta de ar	✓	✗	*SOB*
Dor no abdômen	✓	✗	*ABD Pain*
Ânsia de vômito	✓	✗	*Nausea*
Vômitos	✓	✗	*Vomiting*
Diarreia	✓	✗	*Diarrhea*
Inchaço	✓	✗	*Swelling*
Fraqueza	✓	✗	*New Weakness*

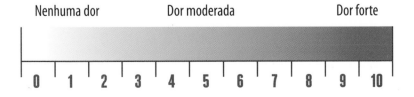
Olá eu sou um profissional da área de saúde. Eu não falo Português.

Hello, I am a healthcare professional. I do not speak Portuguese.

Mostre – me (neste desenho de uma pessoa) onde você sente dores.

Please point (on this picture of a person) to where you have pain.

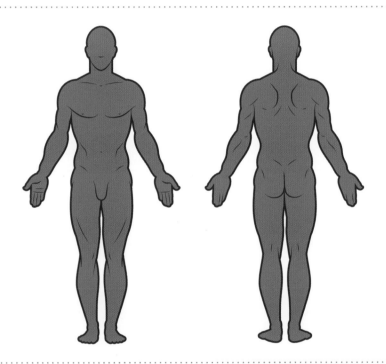

Favor mostrar (nesta tabela) o nível de dor que você está sentindo.

Please point (on this scale) to rate your pain:

Nenhuma dor	Dor moderada	Dor forte

0 1 2 3 4 5 6 7 8 9 10

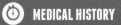
Responda minhas perguntas dizendo sim ou não.

Respond to me only yes or no.   *Do/Have you had:*

Você tem alergia a remédios?	✓	✗	*Rx Allergies*
Você tem asma?	✓	✗	*Asthma*
Você tem um histórico de câncer?	✓	✗	*Hx of Ca*
Você tem insuficiência cardíaca?	✓	✗	*CHF*
Você tem um histórico de insuficiência renal?	✓	✗	*CRF*
Você já teve um infarto?	✓	✗	*CVA*
Você é diabético (a)?	✓	✗	*DM*
Você tem enfisema?	✓	✗	*Emphysema*
Você tem o vírus HIV ou AIDS?	✓	✗	*HIV/AIDS*
Você tem pressão alta?	✓	✗	*HTN*
Você já teve um ataque cardíaco?	✓	✗	*An MI*
Você tem problemas psicológicos?	✓	✗	*Psych Issues*
Você teve uma cirurgia recente?	✓	✗	*Recent Surgery*
Você tem um histórico de convulsões?	✓	✗	*Hx of Sz*

PORTUGUESE / Português

88

Olá, eu sou um profissional da área de saúde. Eu não falo Português.
Hello, I am a healthcare professional. I do not speak Portuguese.

Responda minhas perguntas dizendo sim ou não.
Respond to me only *yes* or *no*.

Você está grávida?	✓	✗	*Are you pregnant?*
Sua bolsa rompeu?	✓	✗	*Has your water broken?*
Você está tendo contrações?	✓	✗	*Are you having contractions?*
O bebê está nascendo agora?	✓	✗	*Is the baby coming now?*
Você tem dor abdominal?	✓	✗	*Do you have ABD pain?*
Você tem dor vaginal?	✓	✗	*Do you have vaginal pain?*
Você está tendo sangramento vaginal?	✓	✗	*Do you have vaginal bleeding?*
Você tem corrimento vaginal?	✓	✗	*Do you have uncommon vaginal discharge?*
A sua gravidez é de alto risco?	✓	✗	*Are you a high-risk pregnancy?*
Você teve uma lesão física recente?	✓	✗	*Have you had a recent physical injury?*
Você já teve complicações com uma gravidez passada?	✓	✗	*Have you had complications with a past pregnancy?*

Indique quantas semanas se passaram desde seu último ciclo menstrual.

Indicate how many weeks have passed since your last menstrual period.

< 1 2 3 4 5 6 7 8 9

Indique há quantos meses você está grávida.

Indicate how many months you have been pregnant.

< 1 2 3 4 5 6 7 8 9

Indique a data em que você deve dar à luz.

Indicate what date you are due to give birth.

Janeiro	Maio	Setembro
January	May	September
Fevereiro	Junho	Outubro
February	June	October
Março	Julho	Novembro
March	July	November
Abril	Agosto	Dezembro
April	August	December

1 2 3 4 5 6 7

8 9 10 11 12 13 14

15 16 17 18 19 20 21

22 23 24 25 26 27 28

29 30 31

Indique quantas vezes ficou grávida.

Indicate how many times you have been pregnant.

0 1 2 3 4 5 6 7 8 9

Indique quantos filhos você tem.

Indicate how many children you have.

0 1 2 3 4 5 6 7 8 9

Indique quantos abortamentos (espontâneos ou não) você teve.

Indicate how many abortions or miscarriages you have had.

0 1 2 3 4 5 6 7 8 9

PORTUGUESE / Português

Um tradutor estará aqui em breve.
An interpreter will be here shortly.

Faça o favor de urinar neste recipiente.
Quando você terminar, por favor, coloque a tampa e dê o recipiente para mim.
Please urinate in this cup. When you are finished, please attach the lid.

Eu preciso colocar o soro. Isso pode doer um pouco.
I need to start an IV. This may hurt a little.

Eu preciso colocar alguns adesivos em seu peito, para examinar seu coração.
I need to put some stickers on your chest in order to examine your heart.

Eu preciso colocar um tubo em sua bexiga. Será um pouco desconfortável.
I need to put a tube in your bladder. This will be uncomfortable.

Eu preciso examinar sua cabeça e rosto.
I need to examine your head and face.

Por favor, abra sua boca.
Please open your mouth.

Eu preciso examinar seu peito, coração e pulmões.
I need to examine your chest, heart, and lungs.

Preciso examinar seu abdomen. Isto pode ser desconfortável.
I need to examine your abdomen. Slight discomfort may occur.

Preciso examinar sua pelve e o reto. Isto pode ser desconfortável.
I need to examine your pelvis and rectum. Slight discomfort may occur.

Eu vou lhe uma medicação que pode fazê-lo sentir-se temporariamente desconfortável.
I am going to give you a medication that may cause temporary discomfort.

Eu vou lhe dar uma medicação que pode fazê-lo sentir-se temporariamente sonolento ou tonto.
I am going to give you a medication that may make you feel sleepy or light-headed.

Farei uma tomografia em você. Não vai doer.
I am going to take you to get a medical scan. This will not hurt.

Здравствуйте, я медицинский специалист. Я не говорю по-русски.
Hello, I am a healthcare professional. I do not speak Russian.

Отвечайте мне только да или нет.
Respond to me only *yes* or *no*.

Жалуетесь ли вы на?
Do you have?

Русский	✓	✗	English
головную боль			*A Headache*
головокружение			*Dizziness*
высокую температуру			*A Fever*
боль в груди			*Chest Pain*
одышку			*SOB*
боли в животе			*ABD Pain*
тошноту			*Nausea*
рвоту			*Vomiting*
понос			*Diarrhea*
опухоль			*Swelling*
неожиданную слабость			*New Weakness*

RUSSIAN / Русский

92

Здравствуйте, я медицинский специалист. Я не говорю по-русски.
Hello, I am a healthcare professional. I do not speak Russian.

Пожалуйста, покажите (на этом изображении человека), где болит.
Please point (on this picture of a person) to where you have pain.

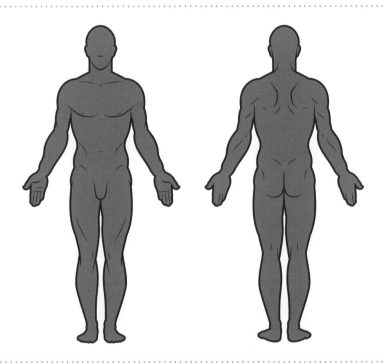

Пожалуйста, укажите (по данной шкале) степень боли.
Please point (on this scale) to rate your pain.

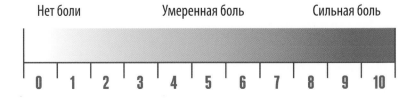

Нет боли   Умеренная боль   Сильная боль

0 1 2 3 4 5 6 7 8 9 10

Отвечайте мне только да или нет.
Respond to me only *yes* or *no*.

Do/Have you had:

Question	✓	✗	English
Есть ли у вас аллергия на медикаменты?	✓	✗	*Rx Allergies*
Есть ли у вас астма?	✓	✗	*Asthma*
Был ли у вас когда-нибудь рак?	✓	✗	*Hx of Ca*
Есть ли у вас застойная сердечная недостаточность?	✓	✗	*CHF*
Была ли у вас когда-нибудь почечная недостаточность?	✓	✗	*CRF*
Был ли у вас когда-нибудь инсульт?	✓	✗	*CVA*
Есть ли у вас диабет?	✓	✗	*DM*
Есть ли у вас эмфизема?	✓	✗	*Emphysema*
Есть ли у вас ВИЧ или СПИД?	✓	✗	*HIV/AIDS*
У вас высокое артериальное давление?	✓	✗	*HTN*
Был ли у вас когда-нибудь сердечный приступ?	✓	✗	*An MI*
Есть ли у вас психологические проблемы?	✓	✗	*Psych Issues*
Переносили ли вы операцию в недавнем времени?	✓	✗	*Recent Surgery*
Были ли у вас когда-нибудь судорожные припадки?	✓	✗	*Hx of Sz*

RUSSIAN / Русский

94

Здравствуйте, я медицинский специалист. Я не говорю по-русски.
Hello, I am a healthcare professional. I do not speak Russian.

Отвечайте мне только да или нет.
Respond to me only *yes* or *no*.

Вы беременны?	✓ ✗	Are you pregnant?
Отошли ли у вас воды?	✓ ✗	Has your water broken?
У вас есть схватки?	✓ ✗	Are you having contractions?
Ребенок выходит?	✓ ✗	Is the baby coming now?
Есть ли у вас боль в животе?	✓ ✗	Do you have ABD pain?
Есть ли у вас влагалищные боли?	✓ ✗	Do you have vaginal pain?
У вас есть влагалищное кровотечение?	✓ ✗	Do you have vaginal bleeding?
Есть ли у вас необычные влагалищные выделения?	✓ ✗	Do you have uncommon vaginal discharge?
Входит ли ваша беременность в группу риска?	✓ ✗	Are you a high-risk pregnancy?
Была ли у вас недавняя физическая травма?	✓ ✗	Have you had a recent physical injury?
Были ли у вас осложнения при последней беременности?	✓ ✗	Have you had complications with a past pregnancy?

Укажите, сколько недель прошло со времени последнего менструального цикла.

Indicate how many weeks have passed since your last menstrual period.

<   1   2   3   4   5   6   7   8   9

Укажите, сколько месяцев вы беременны.

Indicate how many months you have been pregnant.

<   1   2   3   4   5   6   7   8   9

Укажите ожидаемую дату родов.

Indicate the date you are due to give birth.

Январь January	Май May	Сентябрь September
Февраль February	Июнь June	Октябрь October
Март March	Июль July	Ноябрь November
Апрель April	Август August	Декабрь December

1   2   3   4   5   6   7

8   9   10   11   12   13   14

15   16   17   18   19   20   21

22   23   24   25   26   27   28

29   30   31

Укажите, сколько раз вы были беременны.

Indicate how many times you have been pregnant.

0   1   2   3   4   5   6   7   8   9

Укажите, сколько у вас детей.

Indicate how many children you have.

0   1   2   3   4   5   6   7   8   9

Укажите, сколько абортов или выкидышей у вас было.

Indicate how many abortions or miscarriages you have had.

0   1   2   3   4   5   6   7   8   9

Переводчик скоро прибудет.
An interpreter will be here shortly.

Пожалуйста, помочитесь в баночку. Когда закончите, закройте баночку крышкой и дайте её мне.
Please urinate in this cup. When you are finished, please attach the lid.

Мне нужно поставить вам капельницу. Может быть немного больно.
I need to start an IV. This may hurt a little.

Мне нужно прикрепить вам на грудь наклейки, чтобы проверить сердце.
I need to put some stickers on your chest in order to examine your heart.

Мне нужно поставить трубочку вам в мочевой пузырь. Это вызовет дискомфорт.
I need to put a tube in your bladder. This will be uncomfortable.

Мне нужно осмотреть ваши голову и лицо.
I need to examine your head and face.

Пожалуйста, откройте рот.
Please open your mouth.

Мне нужно проверить грудь, сердце и легкие.
I need to examine your chest, heart, and lungs.

Мне нужно проверить ваш живот. Это может быть неприятно.
I need to examine your abdomen. Slight discomfort may occur.

Мне нужно проверить ваш таз и прямую кишку. Это может быть некомфортно.
I need to examine your pelvis and rectum. Slight discomfort may occur.

Сейчас я вам дам лекарство, которое может вызвать у вас временный дискомфорт.
I am going to give you a medication that may cause temporary discomfort.

Сейчас я вам дам препарат, который может вызвать у вас чувство временной сонливости или головокружение.
I am going to give you a medication that may make you feel sleepy or light-headed.

Я направляю вас на лучевое исследование. Это не вызовет боли.
I am going to take you to get a medical scan. This will not hurt.

Hola, soy un(a) profesional de la salud. No hablo Español.
Hello, I am a healthcare professional. I do not speak Spanish.

Respóndame solo sí o no.
Respond to me only *yes* or *no*.

¿Tiene usted?
Do you have?

Dolor de cabeza	✓	✗	*A Headache*
Mareos	✓	✗	*Dizziness*
Fiebre	✓	✗	*A Fever*
Dolor de pecho	✓	✗	*Chest Pain*
Dificultad para respirar	✓	✗	*SOB*
Dolor abdominal	✓	✗	*ABD Pain*
Náuseas	✓	✗	*Nausea*
Vómitos	✓	✗	*Vomiting*
Diarrea	✓	✗	*Diarrhea*
Hinchazón	✓	✗	*Swelling*
Síntomas de debilidad que no sentía antes	✓	✗	*New Weakness*

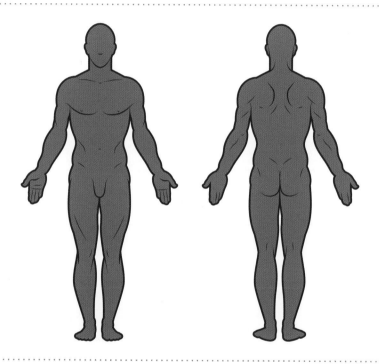
Hola, soy un(a) profesional de la salud. No hablo Español.

Hello, I am a healthcare professional. I do not speak Spanish.

Por favor señale (en esta foto de una persona) donde tiene dolor.

Please point (on this picture of a person) to where you have pain.

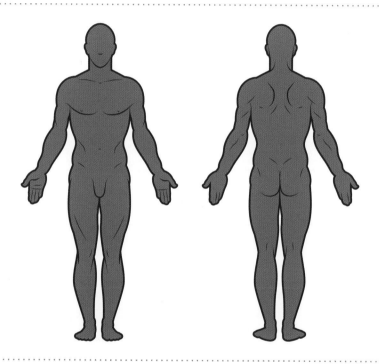

Por favor, indique (en la siguiente escala) la intensidad de su dolor.

Please point (on this scale) to rate your pain.

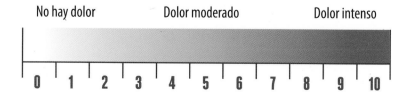

No hay dolor   Dolor moderado   Dolor intenso

0   1   2   3   4   5   6   7   8   9   10

Respóndame solo sí o no.
Respond to me only *yes* or *no*.

Do/Have you had:

¿Tiene alergia a algún medicamento?	✓	✗	*Rx Allergies?*
¿Tiene asma?	✓	✗	*Asthma?*
¿Tiene antecedentes de cáncer?	✓	✗	*Hx of Ca?*
¿Tiene insuficiencia cardiaca congestiva?	✓	✗	*CHF?*
¿Tiene antecedentes de insuficiencia renal?	✓	✗	*CRF?*
¿Ha tenido alguna vez un derrame cerebral?	✓	✗	*CVA?*
¿Tiene diabetes?	✓	✗	*DM?*
¿Tiene enfisema?	✓	✗	*Emphysema?*
¿Tiene VIH o SIDA?	✓	✗	*HIV/AIDS?*
¿Tiene presión arterial alta?	✓	✗	*HTN?*
¿Ha tenido un infarto?	✓	✗	*An MI?*
¿Tiene problemas psicológicos?	✓	✗	*Psych Issues*
¿Se ha sometido recientemente a una cirugía?	✓	✗	*Recent Surgery?*
¿Tiene antecedentes de convulsiones?	✓	✗	*Hx of Sz?*

SPANISH / ESPAÑOL

100

Hola, soy un(a) profesional de la salud. No hablo Español.
Hello, I am a healthcare professional. I do not speak Spanish.

Respóndame solo sí o no.
Respond to me only *yes* or *no*.

¿Está embarazada?	✓	✗	Are you pregnant?
¿Se le ha roto la fuente?	✓	✗	Has your water broken?
¿Tiene contracciones?	✓	✗	Are you having contractions?
¿El bebé ya está bajando?	✓	✗	Is the baby coming now?
¿Tiene dolores abdominales?	✓	✗	Do you have ABD pain?
¿Tiene dolores vaginales?	✓	✗	Do you have vaginal pain?
¿Tiene sangrado vaginal?	✓	✗	Do you have vaginal bleeding?
¿Tiene secreción vaginal poco usual?	✓	✗	Do you have uncommon vaginal discharge?
¿Tiene un embarazo de alto riesgo?	✓	✗	Are you a high-risk pregnancy?
¿Ha sufrido recientemente una lesión física?	✓	✗	Have you had a recent physical injury?
¿Ha tenido complicaciones en su último embarazo?	✓	✗	Have you had complications with a past pregnancy?

Indique hace cuántas semanas tuvo su último ciclo menstrual.

Indicate how many weeks have passed since your last menstrual period.

<   1   2   3   4   5   6   7   8   9

Indique cuántas meses de embarazo tiene.

Indicate how many months you have been pregnant.

<   1   2   3   4   5   6   7   8   9

Indique la fecha en que va a dar a luz.

Indicate the date you are due to give birth.

Enero (January)	Mayo (May)	Setiembre (September)	1	2	3	4	5	6	7
Febrero (February)	Junio (June)	Octubre (October)	8	9	10	11	12	13	14
Marzo (March)	Julio (July)	Noviembre (November)	15	16	17	18	19	20	21
Abril (April)	Agosto (August)	Diciembre (December)	22	23	24	25	26	27	28
			29	30	31				

Indique cuántas veces ha estado embarazada.

Indicate how many times you have been pregnant.

0   1   2   3   4   5   6   7   8   9

Indique cuántos hijos tiene.

Indicate how many children you have.

0   1   2   3   4   5   6   7   8   9

Indique cuántos abortos o abortos espontáneos ha tenido.

Indicate how many abortions or miscarriages you have had.

0   1   2   3   4   5   6   7   8   9

En breve vendrá un traductor.
An interpreter will be here shortly.

Por favor, orine en este envase. Cuando termine, tape el envase y entréguemelo.
Please urinate in this cup. When you are finished, please attach the lid.

Debo colocarle una línea intravenosa. Puede dolerle un poco.
I need to start an IV. This may hurt a little.

Debo ponerle unas etiquetas adhesivas en el pecho para poder examinarle el corazón.
I need to put some stickers on your chest in order to examine your heart.

Debo colocarle una sonda en la vejiga. Va a ser un poco incómodo.
I need to put a tube in your bladder. This will be uncomfortable.

Debo examinarle la cabeza y la cara.
I need to examine your head and face.

Abra la boca por favor.
Please open your mouth.

Debo examinarle el pecho, el corazón y los pulmones.
I need to examine your chest, heart, and lungs.

Debo examinarle el abdomen. Puede resultar incómodo.
I need to examine your abdomen. Slight discomfort may occur.

Debo examinarle la pelvis y el recto. Puede resultar incómodo.
I need to examine your pelvis and rectum. Slight discomfort may occur.

Le voy a dar un medicamento que le puede producir una incomodidad pasajera.
I am going to give you a medication that may cause temporary discomfort.

Le voy a dar un medicamento que le puede producir somnolencia o mareos pasajeros.
I am going to give you a medication that may make you feel sleepy or light-headed.

Lo/La voy a llevar para que le hagan un escáner. No le va a causar dolor.
I am going to take you to get a medical scan. This will not hurt.

Kamusta, ako'y isang propesyonal sa pangangalagang pangkalusugan.
Hindi ako nagsasalita ng Tagalog.

Hello, I am a healthcare professional. I do not speak Tagalog.

Sagutin po ako ng oo o hindi lamang.

Respond to me only *yes* or *no*.

Ikaw ba ay may?

Do you have?

Sakit ng ulo	✓	✗	*A Headache*
Pagkahilo	✓	✗	*Dizziness*
Lagnat	✓	✗	*A Fever*
Pananakit ng dibdib	✓	✗	*Chest Pain*
Pangangapos ng paghinga	✓	✗	*SOB*
Pananakit ng tiyan	✓	✗	*ABD Pain*
Pagduduwal	✓	✗	*Nausea*
Pagsusuka	✓	✗	*Vomiting*
Pagtatae	✓	✗	*Diarrhea*
Pamamaga	✓	✗	*Swelling*
Bagong kahinaan	✓	✗	*New Weakness*

TAGALOG / TAGALOG

Kamusta, ako'y isang propesyonal sa pangangalagang pangkalusugan.
Hindi ako nagsasalita ng Tagalog.
Hello, I am a healthcare professional. I do not speak Tagalog.

Pakituro (sa larawang ito ng isang tao) kung saan ka nakakaramdam ng pananakit.
Please point (on this picture of a person) to where you have pain.

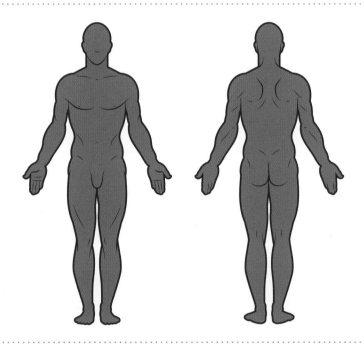

Tumuro (sa scale na ito) upang ilarawan ang nararamdaman mong pananakit.
Please point (on this scale) to rate your pain.

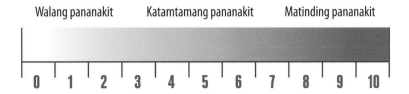

Walang pananakit	Katamtamang pananakit	Matinding pananakit

0 1 2 3 4 5 6 7 8 9 10

Sagutin po ako ng oo o hindi lamang.
Respond to me only yes or no.   *Do/Have you had:*

May mga allergy ka ba sa mga gamot?	✓	✗	*Rx Allergies*
Mayroon ka bang hika?	✓	✗	*Asthma*
May kasaysayan ka ba ng kanser?	✓	✗	*Hx of Ca*
Mayroon ka bang paninikip sa pagpalya ng puso?	✓	✗	*CHF*
May kasaysayan ka ba ng pagpalya ng bato?	✓	✗	*CRF*
Na-stroke ka na ba?	✓	✗	*CVA*
Mayroon ka bang diabetes?	✓	✗	*DM*
Mayroon ka bang emphysema?	✓	✗	*Emphysema*
Mayroon ka bang HIV o AIDs?	✓	✗	*HIV/AIDS*
Mayroon ka bang mataas na presyon ng dugo?	✓	✗	*HTN*
Inatake ka na ba sa puso?	✓	✗	*An MI*
Mayroon ka bang mga problemang pangkaisipan?	✓	✗	*Psych Issues*
Naoperahan ka ba kamakailan?	✓	✗	*Recent Surgery*
Mayroon ka bang kasaysayan ng atake?	✓	✗	*Hx of Sz*

TAGALOG / Tagalog

106

Kamusta, ako'y isang propesyonal sa pangangalagang pangkalusugan. Hindi ako nagsasalita ng Tagalog.

Hello, I am a healthcare professional. I do not speak Tagalog.

Sagutin po ako ng oo o hindi lamang.

Respond to me only *yes* or *no*.

Tagalog	✔	✖	English
Buntis ka ba?			Are you pregnant?
Pumutok na ba ang iyong panubigan?			Has your water broken?
Nagkakaroon ba ng mga paghilab ang iyong tiyan?			Are you having contractions?
Palabas na ba ang sanggol?			Is the baby coming now?
Masakit ba ang iyong tiyan?			Do you have ABD pain?
Masakit ba iyong ari?			Do you have vaginal pain?
Dumudugo ba ang iyong ari?			Do you have vaginal bleeding?
May lumalabas ba sa iyong ari na hindi pangkaraniwan?			Do you have uncommon vaginal discharge?
Malaki ba ang panganib sa iyong pagbubuntis?			Are you a high-risk pregnancy?
Napinsala ba ang iyong katawan kamakailan?			Have you had a recent physical injury?
Nagkaroon ka ba ng mga kumplikasyon sa nakaraang pagbubuntis?			Have you had complications with a past pregnancy?

Ipabatid kung ilang linggo na ang nakalipas mula noong pinakahuli mong regla.
Indicate how many weeks have passed since your last menstrual period.

< 1 2 3 4 5 6 7 8 9

Ipabatid kung ilang buwan ka nang buntis.
Indicate how many months you have been pregnant.

< 1 2 3 4 5 6 7 8 9

Ilagay ang petsa kung kailan ka nakatakdang manganak.
Indicate the date you are due to give birth.

Enero (January)   Mayo (May)   Setyembre (September)
Pebrero (February)   Hunyo (June)   Oktubre (October)
Marso (March)   Hulyo (July)   Nobyembre (November)
Abril (April)   Agosto (August)   Disyembre (December)

1 2 3 4 5 6 7
8 9 10 11 12 13 14
15 16 17 18 19 20 21
22 23 24 25 26 27 28
29 30 31

Ipabatid kung ilang beses ka nang nabuntis.
Indicate how many times you have been pregnant.

0 1 2 3 4 5 6 7 8 9

Ipabatid kung ilan ang inyong mga anak.
Indicate how many children you have.

0 1 2 3 4 5 6 7 8 9

Ipabatid kung ilang beses na kayong dumanas ng aborsiyon o pagkalaglag.
Indicate how many abortions or miscarriages you have had.

0 1 2 3 4 5 6 7 8 9

Malapit nang dumating ang isang interpreter.
An interpreter will be here shortly.

Mangyaring umihi sa cup na ito. Pagkatapos mo, pakilagay ang takip at ibigay sa akin ang cup.
Please urinate in this cup. When you are finished, please attach the lid.

Kailangan kong simulan ang isang IV. Maaari itong sumakit nang kaunti.
I need to start an IV. This may hurt a little.

Kailangan kong maglagay ng ilang sticker sa dibdib mo upang masuri ang iyong puso.
I need to put some stickers on your chest in order to examine your heart.

Kailangan kong maglagay ng tubo sa iyong pantog, Hindi ito magiging komportable.
I need to put a tube in your bladder. This will be uncomfortable.

Kailangan kong suriin ang iyong ulo at mukha.
I need to examine your head and face.

Pakibuka ang iyong bibig.
Please open your mouth.

Kailangan kong suriin ang iyong dibdib, puso, at baga.
I need to examine your chest, heart, and lungs.

Kailangan kong suriin ang iyong tiyan. Ito ay maaaring hindi komportable.
I need to examine your abdomen. Slight discomfort may occur.

Kailangan kong suriin ang iyong balakang at tumbong. Ito ay maaaring hindi komportable.
I need to examine your pelvis and rectum. Slight discomfort may occur.

Bibigyan kita ng gamot kung saan maaari kang pansamantalang hindi maging komportable.
I am going to give you a medication that may cause temporary discomfort.

Bibigyan kita ng gamot kung saan maaari kang antukin o mahilo.
I am going to give you a medication that may make you feel sleepy or light-headed.

Isasailalim kita sa medical scan. Hindi ito masakit.
I am going to take you to get a medical scan. This will not hurt.

السلام علیکم، میں ایک پیشہ ور حفضان صحت مہیا کرنے والا / والی ہوں. میں اردو نہں بولتا / بولتی.

Hello, I am a healthcare professional. I do not speak Urdu.

مجھے صرف ہاں یا نہیں میں جواب دیجیے.

Respond to me only *yes* or *no*.

کیا آپ کو درج ذیل دی گئی علامات میں سے لائق لاہق ہے؟

Do you have?

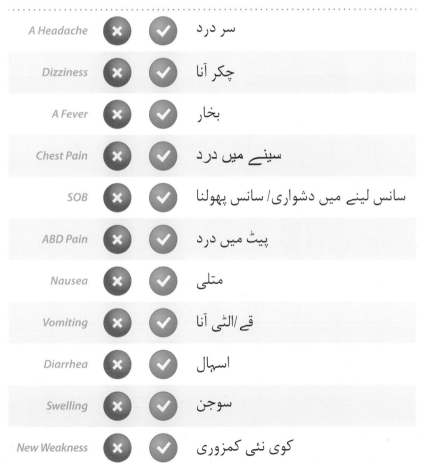

A Headache	✖	✔	سر درد
Dizziness	✖	✔	چکر آنا
A Fever	✖	✔	بخار
Chest Pain	✖	✔	سینے میں درد
SOB	✖	✔	سانس لینے میں دشواری/ سانس پھولنا
ABD Pain	✖	✔	پیٹ میں درد
Nausea	✖	✔	متلی
Vomiting	✖	✔	قے/الٹی آنا
Diarrhea	✖	✔	اسہال
Swelling	✖	✔	سوجن
New Weakness	✖	✔	کوئی نئی کمزوری

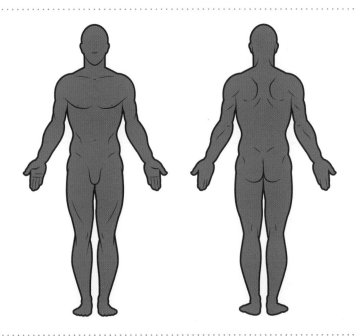
URDU / اردو

السلام علیکم، میں ایک پیشہ ور حفظان صحت مہیا کرنے والا / والی ہوں. میں اردو نہں بولتا / بولتی.

Hello, I am a healthcare professional. I do not speak Urdu.

برائے مہربانی (اس شخص کی تصویر پر) اشارہ کر کہ دکھایں جہاں آپ کو درد ہے.

Please point (on this picture of a person) to where you have pain.

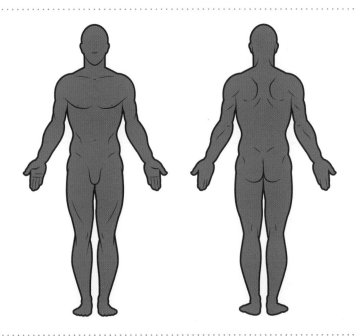

برائے مہربانی پیمانے کی جانب اشارہ کر کہ اپنے درد کی شرح بیان کیجئے.

Please point (on this scale) to rate your pain:

کوئی درد نہیں   معتدل/ ہلکا درد   شدید درد

| 0 | 1 | 2 | 3 | 4 | 5 | 6 | 7 | 8 | 9 | 10 |

مجھے صرف ہاں یا نہیں میں جواب دیجیے.

Do/Have you had: | Respond to me only *yes* or *no.*

Rx Allergies	✗	✓	کیا آپ کو دواؤں سے الرجی ہے؟
Asthma	✗	✓	کیا آپ کو دمہ ہے؟
Hx of Ca	✗	✓	کیا آپ کو ماضی میں کبھی کینسر ہوا ہے؟
CHF	✗	✓	کیا آپ کو امتلائی دورہِ دل کا مرض لاحق ہے؟
CRF	✗	✓	کیا آپ کو ماضی میں گردوں کی ناکامی کا مرض ہوا ہے؟
CVA	✗	✓	کیا آپ کو کبھی فالج ہوا ہے؟
DM	✗	✓	کیا آپ کو ضیابیطس ہے؟
Emphysema	✗	✓	کیا آپ کو نفاخ ہے؟
HIV/AIDS	✗	✓	کیا آپ کو ایچ آئی وی یا ایڈز ہے؟
HTN	✗	✓	کیا آپ کوبلند فشار خون (ہای بلڈپریشر) کی تکلیف ہے؟
An MI	✗	✓	کیا آپ کو کبھی دل کا دورہ پڑا ہے؟
Psych Issues	✗	✓	کیا آپ کسی نفسیاتی مشکلات کا شکار ہیں؟
Recent Surgery	✗	✓	کیا آپ نے حال ہی میں کوئی جراحی/آپریشن کروایا ہے؟
Hx of Sz	✗	✓	کیا آپ کو ماضی میں کبھی دورہ پڑا ہے؟

URDU / اردو

السلام علیکم، میں ایک پیشہ ور حفظانِ صحت مہیا کرنے والا / والی ہوں. میں اردو نہیں بولتا / بولتی.

Hello, I am a healthcare professional. I do not speak Urdu.

مجھے صرف ہاں یا نہیں میں جواب دیجیے.

Respond to me only *yes* or *no*.

Are you pregnant?	✖	✔	کیا آپ حاملہ ہیں؟
Has your water broken?	✖	✔	کیا آپ کا پانی ٹوٹ گیا ہے؟
Are you having contractions?	✖	✔	کیا آپ کے پٹھے سکڑ رہے ہیں؟
Is the baby coming now?	✖	✔	کیا بچہ ابھی پیدا ہو رہا ہے؟
Do you have ABD pain?	✖	✔	کیا آپ کے پیٹ میں درد/تکلیف ہے؟
Do you have vaginal pain?	✖	✔	کیا آپ کی اندام نہانی میں تکلیف ہے؟
Do you have vaginal bleeding?	✖	✔	کیا آپ کی اندام نہانی سے خون جاری ہے؟
Do you have uncommon vaginal discharge?	✖	✔	کیا آپ کی اندام نہانی سے کسی غیرمعمولی مواد کا اخراج ہو رہا ہے؟
Are you a high-risk pregnancy?	✖	✔	کیا آپ کا حمل زیادہ خطرے والا ہے؟
Have you had a recent physical injury?	✖	✔	کیا آپ کو حال ہی میں کوئی جسمانی چوٹ آئی ہے؟
Have you had complications with a past pregnancy?	✖	✔	کیا آپ کو ماضی میں حمل میں کوئی پیچیدگیاں درپیش تھیں؟

نشاندہی کیجیے کہ آپ کے آخری ایام حیض کو کتنے ہفتے گزر چکے ہیں.

Indicate how many weeks have passed since your last menstrual period.

< 1 2 3 4 5 6 7 8 9

نشاندہی کیجیے کہ آپ کتنے مہینوں سے حاملہ ہیں.

Indicate how many months you have been pregnant.

< 1 2 3 4 5 6 7 8 9

بچے کی ولادت کی تاریخ کی نشاندہی کیجیے.

Indicate what date you are due to give birth.

1 2 3 4 5 6 7	ستمبر September	مئ May	جنوری January
8 9 10 11 12 13 14	اکتوبر October	جون June	فروری February
15 16 17 18 19 20 21	نومبر November	جولائی July	مارچ March
22 23 24 25 26 27 28			
29 30 31	دسمبر December	اگست August	اپریل April

نشاندہی کیجیے کہ آپ کتنی بار حاملہ ہو چکی ہیں.

Indicate how many times you have been pregnant.

0 1 2 3 4 5 6 7 8 9

نشاندہی کیجیے کہ آپ نے کتنے بچّوں کو جنم دیا ہے.

Indicate how many children you have delivered.

0 1 2 3 4 5 6 7 8 9

برائے مہربانی نشاندہی کیجیے کہ آپ کے کتنی مرتبہ اسقاط حمل اور حمل ضائع ہوئے ہیں.

Indicate how many abortions or miscarriages you have had.

0 1 2 3 4 5 6 7 8 9

ایک مترجم جلد ہی یہاں آ جائے گا/گی.

An interpreter will be here shortly.

برائے مہربانی اس کپ میں پیشاب کیجیے. جب آپ فارغ ہو جائیں تو ڈھکن لگا کر کپ مجھے دے دیجیے.

Please urinate in this cup. When you are finished, please attach the lid.

اب مجھے آئی وی شروع کرنی ہے. یہ تھوڑا تکلیف دہ ہو سکتا ہے.

I need to start an IV. This may hurt a little.

مجھے آپ کی چھاتی پر کچھ سٹیکرز لگانے ہیں تاکہ میں آپ کے دل کی جانچ کر سکوں.

I need to put some stickers on your chest in order to examine your heart.

مجھے اپ کے مثانے میں نالی لگانی ہے. یہ تھوڑا غیر آرامدہ محسوس ہو سکتا ہے.

I need to put a tube in your bladder. This will be uncomfortable.

مجھے آپ کا سر اور چہرہ جانچ کرنا ہے.

I need to examine your head and face.

اپنا منہ کھولیے.

Please open your mouth.

مجھے آپ کی چھاتی، دل اور پھیپھڑوں کی جانچ کرنی ہے.

I need to examine your chest, heart, and lungs.

مجھے آپ کے پیٹ کی جانچ کرنا ہے یہ تھوڑا غیر آرامدہ ہو سکتا ہے.

I need to examine your abdomen. Slight discomfort may occur.

مجھے آپ کے دھڑ کے نچلے حصے اور مقعد کی جانچ کرنی ہے. یہ تھوڑا غیر آرامدہ ہو سکتا ہے.

I need to examine your pelvis and rectum. Slight discomfort may occur.

میں آپ کو ایک ایسی دوا دوں گا/گی جو آپ کو عارضی طور پر غیر آرامدہ کر سکتی ہے.

I am going to give you a medication that may cause temporary discomfort.

میں آپ کو ایک ایسی دوا دوں گا/گی جس سے آپ عارضی طور پر اپنے آپ ایسا محسوس کریں گے جیسے آپ کو نیند آ رہی ہے یا چکر.

I am going to give you a medication that may make you feel sleepy or light-headed.

میں آپ کو طبی سکین کے لیے لے کر جا رہا/جا رہی ہوں. اس سے آپ کو کوئی تکلیف نہیں ہو گی.

I am going to take you to get a medical scan. This will not hurt.

Chào, tôi là nhân viên y tế chuyên nghiệp. Tôi không nói tiếng Việt.
Hello, I am a healthcare professional. I do not speak Vietnamese.

Chỉ trả lời tôi có hoặc không.
Respond to me only *yes* or *no*.

Quý vị có bị?
Do you have?

đau đầu	✓	✗	*A Headache*
Chóng mặt	✓	✗	*Dizziness*
nóng sốt	✓	✗	*A Fever*
đau ngực	✓	✗	*Chest Pain*
khó thở	✓	✗	*SOB*
đau bụng	✓	✗	*ABD Pain*
Buồn nôn	✓	✗	*Nausea*
nôn mửa	✓	✗	*Vomiting*
Tiêu chảy	✓	✗	*Diarrhea*
Sưng tấy	✓	✗	*Swelling*
Chỗ đau yếu nào mới	✓	✗	*New Weakness*

Chào, tôi là nhân viên y tế chuyên nghiệp. Tôi không nói tiếng Việt.

Hello, I am a healthcare professional. I do not speak Vietnamese.

Vui lòng chỉ (vào tấm hình con người này) chỗ ông/bà đang bị đau.

Please point (on this picture of a person) to where you have pain.

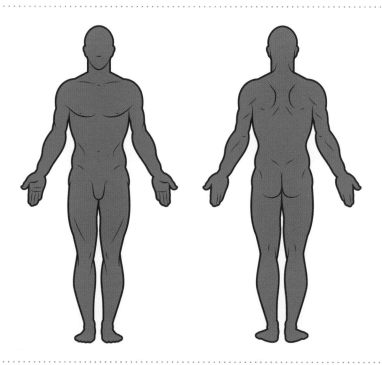

Vui lòng chỉ (vào thang điểm này) để xác định cơn đau của quý vị.

Please point (on this scale) to rate your pain.

Không đau	Đau vừa phải	Đau dữ dội

0 1 2 3 4 5 6 7 8 9 10

Chỉ trả lời tôi có hoặc không.

Respond to me only *yes* or *no*.

Do/Have you had:

Quý vị có bị Dị Ứng với thuốc men không?	✓	✗	*Rx Allergies*
Quý vị có bị bệnh hen suyễn không?	✓	✗	*Asthma*
Quý vị có tiền sử bị bệnh ung thư không?	✓	✗	*Hx of Ca*
Quý vị có bị chứng nhồi máu suy tim không?	✓	✗	*CHF*
Quý vị có tiền sử bị chứng suy thận không?	✓	✗	*CRF*
Quý vị có bao giờ bị đột quỵ không?	✓	✗	*CVA*
Quý vị có bị bệnh tiểu đường không?	✓	✗	*DM*
Quý vị có bị bệnh khí thũng không?	✓	✗	*Emphysema*
Quý vị có bị nhiễm HIV hoặc bệnh AIDs không?	✓	✗	*HIV/AIDS*
Quý vị có bị bệnh cao huyết áp không?	✓	✗	*HTN*
Quý vị có từng bị đau tim không?	✓	✗	*An MI*
Quý vị có bị các vấn đề về tâm lý không?	✓	✗	*Psych Issues*
Quý vị có trải qua ca phẫu thuật nào gần đây không?	✓	✗	*Recent Surgery*
Quý vị có tiền sử lên cơn động kinh không?	✓	✗	*Hx of Sz*

VIETNAMESE / TIẾNG VIỆT

118

Chào, tôi là nhân viên y tế chuyên nghiệp. Tôi không nói tiếng Việt.
Hello, I am a healthcare professional. I do not speak Vietnamese.

Chỉ trả lời tôi có hoặc không.
Respond to me only *yes* or *no*.

Bà đang có thai phải không?			Are you pregnant?
Bà bị vỡ nước ối chưa?			Has your water broken?
Bà đang bị co thắt dạ con phải không?			Are you having contractions?
Đứa bé đang sắp ra bây giờ phải không?			Is the baby coming now?
Bà có bị đau bụng không?			Do you have ABD pain?
Bà có bị đau ở âm đạo không?			Do you have vaginal pain?
Bà có từng bị chảy máu ở âm đạo không?			Do you have vaginal bleeding?
Bà có bị tiết dịch âm đạo bất thường không?			Do you have uncommon vaginal discharge?
Bà thuộc nhóm người mang thai có nguy cơ cao phải không?			Are you a high-risk pregnancy?
Bà có bị chấn thương nào trên cơ thể gần đây không?			Have you had a recent physical injury?
Bà có gặp các khó khăn rắc rối nào trong lần thai nghén trước không?			Have you had complications with a past pregnancy?

Xin cho biết chu kỳ kinh nguyệt trước của bà cách nay được mấy tuãn rồi.
Indicate how many weeks have passed since your last menstrual period.

< 1 2 3 4 5 6 7 8 9

Xin cho biết bà đã có thai được bao nhiêu tháng rồi.
Indicate how many months you have been pregnant.

< 1 2 3 4 5 6 7 8 9

Xin cho biết bà sẽ sanh nở vào ngày tháng nào.
Indicate the date you are due to give birth.

Tháng Giêng January	Tháng Năm May	Tháng Chín September	1 2 3 4 5 6 7
Tháng Hai February	Tháng Sáu June	Tháng Mười October	8 9 10 11 12 13 14
Tháng Ba March	Tháng Bảy July	Tháng Mười Một November	15 16 17 18 19 20 21
Tháng Tư April	Tháng Tám August	Tháng Mười Hai December	22 23 24 25 26 27 28
			29 30 31

Xin cho biết bà đã có thai được bao nhiêu lần rồi.
Indicate how many times you have been pregnant.

0 1 2 3 4 5 6 7 8 9

Xin cho biết bà có được bao nhiêu đứa con.
Indicate how many children you have.

0 1 2 3 4 5 6 7 8 9

Xin cho biết bà đã bị phá thai hoặc bị sẩy thai bao nhiêu lần rồi.
Indicate how many abortions or miscarriages you have had.

0 1 2 3 4 5 6 7 8 9

Thông dịch viên sẽ sớm có mặt tại đây.
An interpreter will be here shortly.

Vui lòng đi tiểu vào trong cốc này. Khi quý vị đi xong, vui lòng đậy nắp lại và đưa cái cốc cho tôi.
Please urinate in this cup. When you are finished, please attach the lid.

Tôi cần đặt ống truyền dịch. Việc này có thể làm quý vị bị nhói đau.
I need to start an IV. This may hurt a little.

Tôi cần đặt vài miếng dán lên trên ngực để khám tim cho quý vị.
I need to put some stickers on your chest in order to examine your heart.

Tôi cần đặt một cái ống vào trong bàng quang. Việc này sẽ làm quý vị khó chịu.
I need to put a tube in your bladder. This will be uncomfortable.

Tôi cần khám đầu và mặt cho quý vị.
I need to examine your head and face.

Vui lòng há miệng ra.
Please open your mouth.

Tôi cần khám ngực, tim và phổi cho quý vị.
I need to examine your chest, heart, and lungs.

Tôi cần khám bụng cho quý vị. Việc này có thể làm quý vị khó chịu.
I need to examine your abdomen. Slight discomfort may occur.

Tôi cần khám xương chậu và trực tràng. Việc này có thể làm quý vị khó chịu.
I need to examine your pelvis and rectum. Slight discomfort may occur.

Tôi sẽ cho quý vị một liều thuốc và nó có thể làm quý vị thấy khó chịu chốc lát.
I am going to give you a medication that may cause temporary discomfort.

Tôi sẽ cho quý vị một liều thuốc và nó có thể làm quý vị cảm thấy buồn ngủ hoặc mơ màng trong chốc lát.
I am going to give you a medication that may make you feel sleepy or light-headed.

Tôi sẽ dẫn quý vị đi chụp hình y khoa. Việc này sẽ không làm quý vị đau.
I am going to take you to get a medical scan. This will not hurt.

ABOUT THE AUTHOR   121

Neil Bobenhouse, MHA, EMT-P

Neil Bobenhouse is a paramedic, entrepreneur, and language enthusiast currently working for the St. Louis City Fire Department. He holds a bachelor's degree in psychology and a master's degree in health administration, both from Saint Louis University. Neil founded Bobenhouse Industries with the vision to create real-world solutions for the healthcare industry.

PHRASEBOOK CONTRIBUTORS

Mark Levine, MD, FACEP
Assistant Professor, Emergency Medicine
Washington University School of Medicine
Barnes-Jewish Hospital
Medical Director of the St. Louis City Fire Department/EMS

Dean C. Meenach, RN, BSN, CEN, CCRN, CPEN, EMT-P
Director of EMS Education, Mineral Area College

Bobenhouse Industries, LLC
P.O. Box 39044
STL, MO 63139

All translations by International Institute of Saint Louis
Language Services

Graphic Design & Illustrations by Ben Gathard
Bottle Rocket Creative, LLC

ACKNOWLEDGMENTS

The St. Louis City Fire Department

Barnes-Jewish Hospital

Andrea Alameda, Shawn Bittle, Guy Jennings, Bhavin Mehta, Doug Randell, Matt Sleet, and Galen Taylor.

Mike Barnes, Mike Beckenholdt, Jheree Coleman, Jack Douglas, Jeff Glorioso, Pam Miller, Ed Monser, Steve Ponzar, Michelle Vaught, and Chris Yacula.

Sarah Barekzai, Byron Beiermann, Jake Flemming, and Will Massanet.